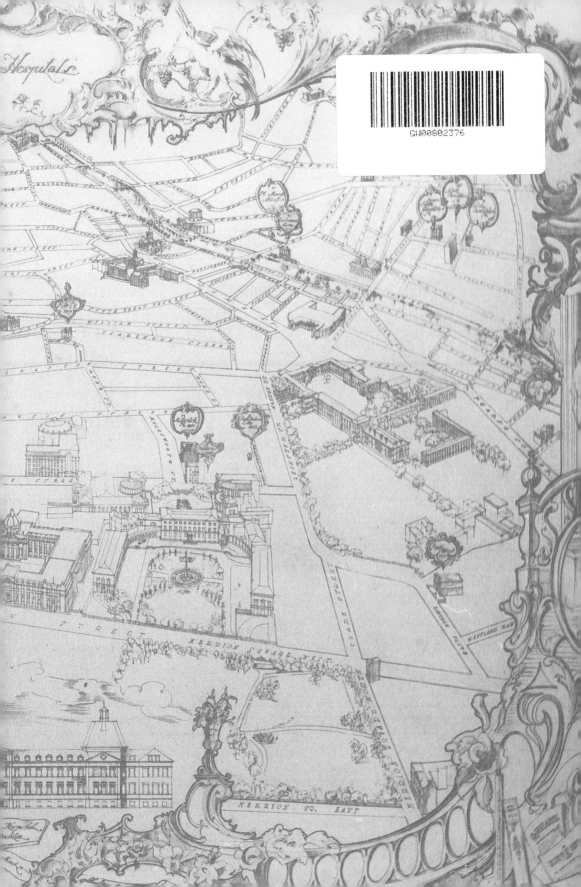

Hospital

DUBLIN'S EYE AND EAR

For Norma

With love from the author

30/3/93

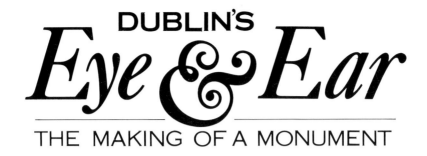

DUBLIN'S
Eye & Ear

THE MAKING OF A MONUMENT

GEAROID CROOKES

Gearoid Crookes

TOWN
HOUSE

Published in 1993 by
Town House and Country House
42 Morehampton Road
Donnybrook
Dublin 4
Ireland

British Library Cataloguing in Publication Data. A catalogue record for this book is available from the British Library

ISBN: 0-948524-57-X

Cover: The Royal Victoria Eye and Ear Hospital, 1992

Managing editor: Treasa Coady
Text editor: Elaine Campion
Cover design: Bill Murphy
Colour origination by the Kulor Centre

Typeset by Printset & Design Ltd, Dublin
Printed in Ireland by Criterion Press, Dublin

*This book is dedicated to the memory
of my dear wife Jean,
of Louis Werner
and Con O'Connell,
loyal colleagues and cherished friends*

CONTENTS

ILLUSTRATIONS

PREFACE

To the President and Council of the Royal Victoria Eye and Ear Hospital, who commissioned the writing of this history, I offer my thanks for the honour of being chosen to do it. For one who has spent much of his working life in the hospital, the task has been not only a labour of love but one of personal enrichment. Liberty of access to the hospital's archive was essential to this production, and I acknowledge being given the facility. Confrontation with two such characters as Wilde and Swanzy, each of giant stature, was something of a historian's dream, and I regret only that considerations of space prevented me from treating them more amply.

The lack of detailed reference to the work of presently active members of staff should be seen as deliberate, with the intention of avoiding invidious mention. The writer esteems the work of all present consultants, many of them his former house officers, with equal admiration, and offers a personal opinion that at no time in its distinguished history has the hospital had available a greater pool of talent than at present. In affectionate remembrance special mention is made of the late Louis Werner, whose interest in the book's early chapters was a source of much encouragement and whose generosity in offering to fund colour reproduction of his father's medical artwork has been loyally sustained by his widow Patricia.

It is axiomatic that where opinions are expressed they are my own. That I suspect they are shared by others remains to be proved, but if any readers feel that my conclusion is worthy of support, it would be well for them to voice their agreement.

Even the Dubliner's affectionate nickname, 'the Eye and Ear', is unduly long for manifold repetition in the pages of a book. As a convention therefore, the abbreviation of RVEEH is routinely used in the text, as well as ENT for the ear, nose and throat specialty, RCSI, TCD, and UCD for the teaching schools, and IOS and OSUK for ophthalmological societies here and in Britain.

The research for this book threw up an amount of historical material which, while not used directly, appeared to be of value. This is attached in the form of appendices.

I extend sincere thanks to the multitude of willing helpers who have assisted in various ways. First among these, Miss Mary St C Tullo was most obliging in furnishing details about her grandfather, Sir Henry Swanzy. The Board of the Adelaide Hospital has kindly permitted reproduction of the portrait painted by Sir Henry's daughter, the artist Mary Swanzy. I am indebted to the entire consultant staff of the Eye and Ear Hospital, past and present, for their help and co-operation, and I ask their forbearance for not naming them individually. I thank Miss A Fitzsimons, matron, Miss E Phelan, assistant matron, and Mr C Huet, nursing tutor, as representatives of the nursing staff; all have been of the greatest assistance. Ms Aida Whyte, hospital registrar, has borne with my requests in and out of season, and among the clerical staff I am particularly obliged to Ms Majella Byrne, Ms Patricia Conn and Ms Christine Hamilton.

To Mrs Isolde den Tonkelaar of the Archive of the University of Utrecht, I am indebted for information about the eye hospital built by Professor Hermann Snellen, together with literature and pictures connected with it. I also thank Dr Peter van de Kemp of UCD for help in translating Dutch text.

It is impossible to overstate the assistance and interest of Hilda O'Connell in a work directly linked with her late father Dr Con O'Connell, my friend of many years. The excellence of Mr Stephen Travers' photographic work proclaims itself to everybody, but his patience with my many requirements was obvious only to me. Dr F O'Siocfrada helped me in dating events and Tony Smith in computer crises. Martin Molony has given invaluable assistance in numerous ways, not least through repeated production of working copies in the course of many revisions, as well as in his vast knowledge of computers, and his sister Patricia helped with the indexing. Paddy O'Callaghan contributed a colourful memoir from the ENT Department of long ago.

Finally, I acknowledge the assistance of my publishers, Town House and Country House, where the expertise and suggestions of Treasa Coady and Elaine Campion came as a light amid darkness. I thank them all sincerely.

Gearoid Crookes

Dublin, 1992

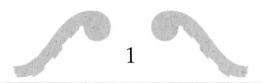

1

THE DAWN OF NECESSITY

In Ireland and England, what is known as the voluntary hospital was not found prior to the eighteenth century. Ireland indeed was, by a short head, enabled to lay claim to the earliest foundation of the kind in the two islands. The Charitable Infirmary, later to be known as Jervis Street Hospital, and today subsumed into the massive foundation of Beaumont Hospital, was started by six Dublin surgeons in Cook Street in 1718. Only in the following year was Britain's first voluntary hospital, the Westminster, opened in London. These originals were soon to be followed by others in both countries.

Despite the distinction bestowed on it by these 'firsts', the eighteenth century, the era of the Enlightenment, is better viewed as a nursery of what was to come. Acting as a hothouse for human thought, it produced the enhanced growth of philanthropic activity that came to full bloom in the next century. Early in the latter can be discerned the first delicate roots of what would eventually become the Royal Victoria Eye and Ear Hospital in Dublin.

By 1800, ophthalmology already had a growing documentation in Europe as a surgical science. The Frenchman Daviel had described the operation for cataract in 1750, and in close association was the Limerick-born Sylvester O'Halloran, who had written about the disorder in 1749 and

1

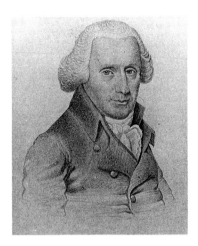

1.1 *Sylvester O'Halloran
(1728-1807), the first Irish
practitioner of cataract extraction.*

was to recur to it at various times in a crowded professional career. The Vienna School of Ophthalmology had been founded by the Empress Maria Theresa in 1775, and accounts of the work of its earliest surgeons, Barth and Beer, were by now filtering abroad. A Europe physically echoing to the strains of the Marseillaise and intellectually quickened by the new ideas of the French Revolution was soon to resound to the tramp of Napoleon's armies, the factor which more than anything would galvanise change in the new century. The time was ripe for progress beyond quack surgery, such as that of the 'Chevalier Taylor, Ophthalmiator' who had toured England and Europe for some fifty years selling salves and performing the unsound, and often blinding, operation of 'couching' cataracts.

With the dawn of the new century there was little longer to wait for the initiatives it promised. Napoleon's imperial progress had led to the Egyptian Campaign (1798-1801) in which thousands of Europeans were drawn to fight and die in North Africa, with many more fated to return home suffering from the dreaded and contagious Egyptian Ophthalmia, a synonym for trachoma. With the spread of this, no longer was eye disease sporadic or even endemic; given the hygiene of the time it bade fair to become epidemic so that, in counteraction, a response from society became necessary. Thus, almost imperceptibly, the search for knowledge changed gear from the passive pursuit of truth to the active search for remedy still enduring to the present day.

Hard upon the Egyptian Campaign, the year 1804 saw the foundation

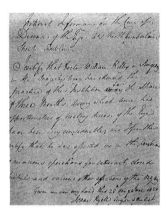

1.2 *Certificate given by Isaac Ryall in
1820. The first known Ophthalmic
Certificate to be issued in Ireland.*

in England of Moorfields, the Royal London Ophthalmic Hospital. Ten
years later there arose in Dublin the National Eye and Ear Infirmary which
could subsequently boast that of the thirty-four ophthalmic hospitals in
Great Britain and Ireland there were only four of earlier date. The four
were those in London (Moorfields, 1804), Exeter (1808), Bristol (1810), and
Bath (1811). The Dublin Infirmary was coeval with that in Manchester,
both being founded in 1814.

Though scanty, the surviving early records of the National help to
clothe the bare fact of its origin. The patron on foundation was the Earl of
Whitworth, then Lord Lieutenant, while the first president was Mr
(afterwards Sir Robert) Peel. At that time Chief Secretary for Ireland, Peel is
better remembered for the eponymous distinction deriving from his later
foundation of the force known to England as the 'bobbies' but which
Ireland called the 'peelers'. Medically, credit as prime mover in setting up
the infirmary goes to a naval doctor, Commander Isaac Ryall, stationed in
Dublin from 1814 to 1827.

Mystery surrounds the circumstances of his becoming Founding Father,
mystery all the deeper in that he achieved the distinction within a month
or two of his arrival in Dublin. Since he had no previous repute for skill or
interest in ophthalmology, and as already for a year another aspirant to the
founding of an eye hospital had been active in Dublin, the existence of
some concealed influence favouring Ryall is to be inferred. The fact of his
being a serving officer can only have been to his advantage, but for lack of
documentation his channel of preferment remains obscure.

Ryall was stationed in Dublin from 1814 to 1827, and however he may have first gained influence, it is certain that, knowing the right people, he nurtured the connection. A letter of 1815 indicates that the Lord Lieutenant was by then his patron; in later proof stands an entry of 1822 noting his appointment as State oculist, an office of dignity though of duties unstated. A document dated 1820 shows him in a teaching role for young naval doctors, one of whom had assisted him in the performance of numerous operations for cataract and other eye conditions.

In the manner of the time, his newborn hospital lacked a permanent home; it is accorded at least three different addresses during his sojourn in Ireland, first at No 10 St Mary's Abbey, later successively in Northumberland and Gloucester Streets. At the least he must have run it with personal capability, for when the Navy recalled him to England the reported result was that '....the Institution fell to the ground, it being held in a house rented by him, which of course was given up'. The odd phrasing happily did not refer to a physical collapse, but to the lack of what we would today call infrastructure. Absence of the hospital amenity was quickly recognised and a committee was formed which in 1829 solicited the attendance of the Lord Lieutenant, the Duke of Northumberland, at a charity sermon in aid of the institution. His Grace replied that having a particular objection to charity sermons he proposed as an alternative the holding of a ball, which he promised to support. The duke's frank preference for a party led to a happy outcome in 1830 when a May Day Ball earned £600 for the infirmary.

Ryall's infirmary was the earliest progenitor of the twentieth-century Eye and Ear Hospital, to which it therefore contributed the priceless gift of ancient lineage. Before coming to the ultimate metamorphosis, a review of other nineteenth-century ophthalmic foundations in Dublin shows that from this first one in 1814 to the last in 1872 there were seven such institutions active at various times, though most of them for brief periods. Their overlappings and extinctions can be tabulated as follows:

The National Eye Hospital	1814-97
Institute for the Cure of Diseases of the Eye	1817-23
St Mary's Hospital and Dublin's Eye Infirmary	1819-31
The Ophthalmic Hospital	1829-34
The Coombe Lying-in Hospital and Dublin Ophthalmic Dispensary	1836-47
St Mark's Ophthalmic Hospital for Diseases of the Eye and Ear	1844-97
Dublin Infirmary for Diseases of the Eye and Ear	1872-75
Royal Victoria Eye and Ear Hospital	1897 to date

It can be seen that five of these were short-lived, so short indeed that present lack of documentation makes it difficult to do more than enumerate them. However, we know at least that two of the five were founded by Arthur Jacob, that irascible genius who, despite an abiding interest in ophthalmology, failed to secure for his ophthalmic offspring the durability achieved in Baggot Street Hospital, whereof he was a co-founder.

Jacob's two eye hospitals were the Institute for the Cure of Diseases of the Eye (1817-23) and the Ophthalmic Hospital (1829-34). In between there rose and fell the curiously named St Mary's Hospital and Dublin's Eye Infirmary. With its twelve years in existence (1819-31) this had the longest life span of the five ephemeral foundations. Thanks to the archaeological industry of the late L B Somerville-Large, we have a drawing of the building it occupied at 36 Lower Ormond Quay (see Plate 2).

The fourth of the five was associated with the Coombe Lying-in Hospital. Lasting eleven years, it was clearly an annexe to the main business of the establishment, succumbing to the terrible pressures of the late 1840s when famine stalked the land.

The last transient was a late arrival, situated at 23 Ely Place from 1872 to 1875. Founded by Archibald Hamilton Jacob, son of the more famous Arthur, and called the Dublin Infirmary for Diseases of the Eye and Ear, a vivid picture survives in Somerville-Large's account of it: 'No 23 Ely Place was the house where Jacob was born, where he had come to join his father in ophthalmic practice and where after his father had retired to England in 1869, he had come to live himself. It is a large brick-faced, four-storied Georgian house, but its capacity must then have been strained to the utmost. The in-patient accommodation was "eighteen beds for poor persons besides pay-patients"; there was an operating theatre; the extern dispensary was held three mornings a week at 9.30, and one must presume also that Jacob carried on his private consulting work there. This house also served as the offices of both the *Medical Press and Circular* and the *Irish Medical Directory*, both of which Jacob edited. Jacob was a married man, and was ultimately to have twelve children, some of whom were already born. In these circumstances and taking into consideration the nursing and domestic staffs required, also the housing of "a resident secretary", we need hardly wonder that this hospital only lasted three years. It is doubtful if a consultant's wife in Dublin now would tolerate it for three days.'

Thus in 1875 there remained two hardy survivors, already standing to one another in a state of competition that would become increasingly hard to justify. These were Ryall's National Eye Hospital founded in 1814, and St Mark's Ophthalmic Hospital for Diseases of the Eye and Ear, founded by William Wilde in 1844. It will next be necessary to trace the fortunes of each up to their coalescence into a single establishment, a union giving birth to the Royal Victoria Eye and Ear Hospital in 1897.

While many names are associated with the genesis and growth of these several hospitals, their story is pre-eminently that of their two remarkable founders, William Wilde and Henry Swanzy. With careers overlapping by a few short years, in the circumscribed society of their time a meeting between them would have been inevitable, though it went unrecorded. This is regrettable, for such conjunction of two giants held the bones of history. Each had the quality of greatness, which has many guises, among which tolerance of one's rivals is no certain concomitant. The identification of this talent of greatness in two such differing characters will occupy us for the next few chapters.

1.3 *(Opposite) Sir Henry Swanzy, 1844-1913*

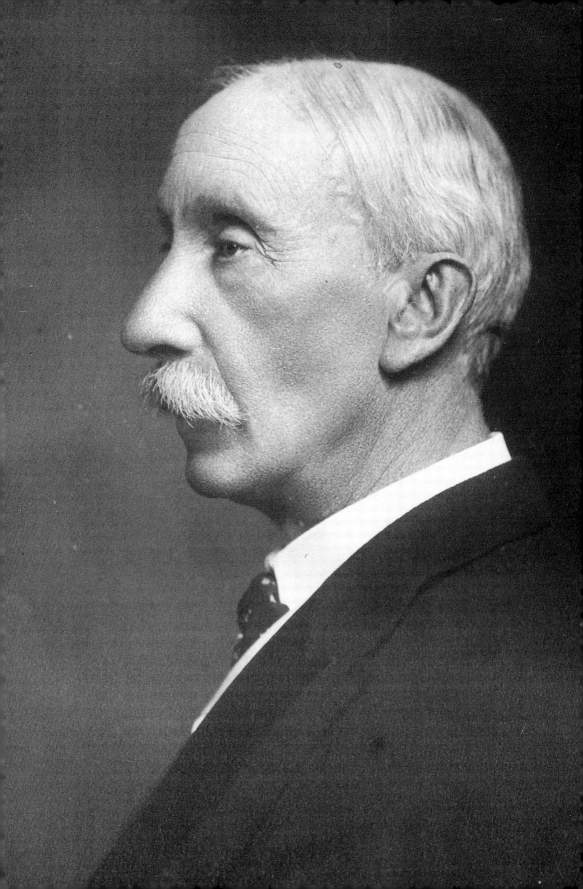

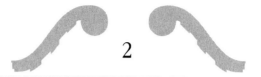

2

A VERSATILE FOUNDER

Following convenience rather than strict chronology, it is easier to deal first with St Mark's Hospital, founded by William Wilde in 1844, in succession to his earlier Dispensary for Eye Diseases. Even though Ryall's foundation was earlier in time, St Mark's, with roots dating closer to the present age, has a history less chequered than that of the National Eye Infirmary, and therefore easier to grasp. Above all, the documentation is profuse and exact, compatible with its founder's gift for classification.

William Wilde, the product of mixed Irish and English stock, was born near Castlerea in County Roscommon in 1815. Son of the local doctor, he showed early aptitude for historical and antiquarian studies and was fluent in both Irish and English. Being destined to follow his father's career, he was sent for schooling to the Royal School, Banagher, and later to the Diocesan School at Elphin. In 1832 he arrived in Dublin to commence training in surgery at Dr Steevens' Hospital, where among his mentors were Abraham Colles and William Stokes. At that time private medical schools were common, and to supplement the practical experience of hospital, Wilde chose to attend Surgeon Cusack's popular Park Street School of Medicine, in premises adjoining the back gate of Trinity College. In those days he can have little foreseen how his later destiny would link him with this building.

After four years he satisfied his teachers and was granted Letters Testimonial from the Royal College of Surgeons. At this point Fortune smiled, in providing a wealthy patient needing a personal medical attendant to act also as travelling companion. The patient's name was Robert Meiklam, who may have belonged to one of the several families of that name then to be found in Glasgow. There is no record of his complaint; perhaps it was tuberculosis, since his ability to move around was uninhibited. The important thing was that he owned a private steam yacht, the *Crusader,* and was Wilde's counterpart in having an omnivorous curiosity. The prospect offered by such an opportunity was life-enhancing and the young Dublin doctor grasped it eagerly.

Wilde was in fact a near-genius, and this journey, taken somewhat like the Grand Tour had been a century before, was his proving ground. The circuit led to Portugal, the Canaries, Gibraltar, Algiers, Malta, Egypt and the Holy Land, an itinerary sufficient to prompt a host of questions. Wilde asked them all and on his return was to describe his experiences in a book entitled *Narrative of a Voyage,* which helped in financing the years to follow.

Back in Dublin, with a view to starting practice, he took rooms at 195 Great Brunswick Street, now Pearse Street. During this period he also found time to prepare scientific papers, as well as lectures for delivery to learned bodies like the Royal Irish Academy in Dublin and to a meeting of the British Association which he attended in Birmingham. Through the former he met George Petrie, the great archaeologist, and William Rowan Hamilton, the future discoverer of quaternions. With these men of weight in the intellectual establishment he was to make lasting friendships.

It is evident from all of this that the young man of twenty-three, waiting for patients in Brunswick Street, was something of a caged eagle eager to fly. He was not without options. In the light of his literary success he could take to literature, as his friend and medical colleague Charles Lever was shortly to do; alternatively he could concentrate on his scientific researches, which had been well received at the British Association; lastly he could pursue the career of medicine he had trained for. He chose the latter and decided to use the £250 he received for his book to help in paying for postgraduate studies in diseases of the eye and ear.

This decision had certainly been influenced by what he had seen of the prevalence of trachoma in Egypt. This ophthalmic disease, which flourished in conditions of dirt and overcrowding, was widespread in the nineteenth century, when it was reliably claimed that, world-wide, it was the greatest single cause of blindness. Indeed, a prominent reservoir of

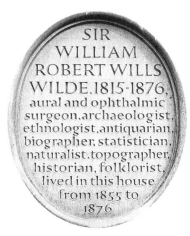

2.1 *Plaque commemorating Sir William Wilde at his residence in No 1 Merrion Square.*

infection existed among the poor in Ireland, leading to recurrent epidemics. In Egypt however it was not merely epidemic, but pandemic, resultant on a teeming population living in squalor, amid heat, dust, and flies, and with no effective treatment or prophylaxis being available. While he was there Wilde must have seen thousands of blind beggars importuning baksheesh from the prosperous, leading him to recall the problem he remembered in Ireland. And indeed, between the two scenes a military connection existed, the soldier during the Napoleonic Wars being vector of what is now known to be the trachoma virus. Since the trade of soldiering was indigenous to the Irishman, it too often meant that in taking the King's shilling, poor Paddy unwittingly took the infection as well, and worse still, brought it home to a crowded cabin offering ideal conditions for its propagation. Thus the Egyptian experience may well have been the signpost to Wilde's calling.

Medical practice of the nineteenth century required no academic qualification to show particular proficiency in diseases of the special senses, and it was seen as natural for eye and ear conditions to be dealt with by the same individual, trained in the principles of surgery but otherwise guided by the extent of his experience. Certainly some continental university teachers made reputations based on expertise in one or other department of sensory defect; seldom however was one to be found whom today's oculists and aurists would both claim for their own. Wilde was to prove himself one such, along with distinction in other fields.

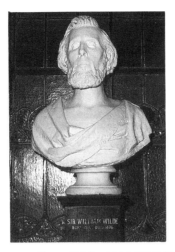

2.2 *Sir William Wilde, 1815-1876 (from the bust in the Royal Victoria Eye and Ear Hospital).*

He was a true polymath, and the plaque to his memory on No 1 Merrion Square celebrates him as 'aural and ophthalmic surgeon, archaeologist, ethnologist, antiquarian, biographer, statistician, naturalist, topographer, historian and folklorist'.

This then was the future image of the young man who left Dublin for London and Vienna in 1840. In the former his goal was Moorfields, in the latter the Allgemeine Krankenhaus, or General Hospital. Moorfields had been founded in 1804 as the London Dispensary for Curing Diseases of the Eye and Ear. Having undergone various changes of site and title, it was now located at its definitive site at Moorfields in the City Road, where it was, and is, known as the Royal London Ophthalmic Hospital. John Saunders, the founder, had been largely impelled by the flood of trachoma cases reaching England after the British evacuation of Egypt in 1803. In its very title his original foundation envisioned care for diseases of both sight and hearing, but for whatever reason, he soon ceased to accept ear cases and concentrated on development of the eye hospital. As T G Wilson, himself an ENT surgeon, has pointed out, this decision had an unexpected side effect, for in jettisoning the aural component Saunders had bequeathed an almost completely unexplored field of research to others. 'Wilde saw this and profited by it, and eventually became the first, and in many ways the greatest of English-speaking ear surgeons.'

Thus simply is explained the genesis of Wilde's role as an ear surgeon. He was to attain an unexampled fame in this specialty, both as operator

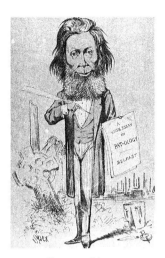

2.3 *Sir William Wilde, a caricature
captioned 'A Wilde (K)night in Ireland's Eye'.*

and teacher. When he first embraced it, it was the field of quackery and superstition; a prevalent remedy for a discharging ear is cited as having been to insert some wool from the left forefoot of a black ram. Wilde resolved to make a basic approach to the subject by working from the principles of pathology, and by reducing treatment to recognised rules of contemporary therapeutics and scientific surgery. In time he was to write a textbook entitled *Aural Surgery,* which remained a standard work for many years, not only in the English-speaking world, but translated, in Austria and Germany as well.

Wilde attended Moorfields for some months, observing the surgical techniques used in cataract removal and the limited number of other eye operations then extant. Trachoma there was in plenty, together with other external diseases, but as Helmholtz had yet to invent the ophthalmoscope, the vast field of medical ophthalmology was still in the future. His next stop was in Vienna, in a sense the hub of nineteenth-century ophthalmology. In the vast General Hospital with over two thousand beds and the nearby Josephinum Academy, were two eye surgeons of merit, Doctors Rosas and Jaeger, under whom he completed his training. By utilising the opportunity of further local travel, he rounded out his education in observation of a lifestyle different from his own, and thus equipped returned to Dublin.

Wilde's biographers have been liberal in reference to his faults as well as his brilliance; beside them both it is but justice to stress his humanity, evident in warm fellow-feeling for those less fortunate than himself. How else to explain the opening of his first dispensary for eye and ear diseases? Aged twenty-six in 1841, he was barely back from his journeyings when his perceived needs of the poor prompted him to this philanthropic exercise.

The first clinic was indeed tentative, opened in a rented stable in Frederick Lane at the rear of a friend's house in Molesworth Street. This dentist friend was Dr Wrigley Grimshaw FRCS who was to feature as consultant surgeon-dentist to Wilde's hospital till 1847. True, the stay in these premises was brief, and the care provided was such as could only be given in a dispensary. In a few years the number of patients so far exceeded expectation, that Wilde was forced to seek expansion, finding fresh quarters close to his own new house in Westland Row. In nearby Mark Street (named after the adjacent Church of St Mark, which, secularised, still stands on Pearse Street) stood the building of an almost extinct surgical institution. Having acquired the tenancy, Wilde moved his infirmary there in 1844, naming it St Mark's Hospital.

The old hospital to which he moved had a complex history. Dating from 1745 and first known as St Nicholas's Hospital or the New Charitable Infirmary, it had become redundant in the Liberties, undergoing transfer to St Mark's parish where it became the United Hospital of St Mark and St Anne. There over the years it had declined, but the organisational structure remained intact, and this was sufficient for its new proprietor, who in addition to refurbishing it, secured revision of its endowment.

It seems clear that the Charitable Commissioners made funds and all available to Wilde, so that by making this coup he doubly benefited his hospital both as to premises and funding. There was another advantage in that he now could point to roots in an older foundation: the historian in him would perceive that by adopting the St Mark invocation he laid claim to the earlier heritage. (A detailed history of this appears as Appendix A.)

In its first year St Mark's had over two thousand out-patients and fifty-seven interns, with an average stay of twenty-four days each. It flourished from the start and the apologia for its existence, published in the first hospital report, runs: 'The want of such an establishment has long been felt by the poor and is generally acknowledged by the upper ranks of society. That such an institution is necessary, we learn from the fact of there being now an ophthalmic or an aural hospital, or both combined, in most of the large towns of England and the continent.'

From 1841 on, Wilde's training and energy made him medically pre-eminent not only in Dublin but increasingly in the wider world also. His

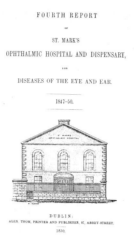

FOURTH REPORT

OF

ST. MARK'S

OPHTHALMIC HOSPITAL AND DISPENSARY,

FOR

DISEASES OF THE EYE AND EAR.

1847-50.

DUBLIN:
ALEX. THOM, PRINTER AND PUBLISHER, 87, ABBEY-STREET.
1850.

2.4 *Cover illustration for Wilde's hospital report on the transfer to the Lincoln Place premises in 1850. Erected for use as a medical school, this building was designed in the form of a Methodist chapel, to which it could be adapted if the medical school failed. It is now owned and used by TCD.*

non-medical activities as antiquary and census commissioner further enhanced his image as a public figure and gained useful publicity for his hospital. This was now co-existing with the National Eye and Ear Infirmary, established in Cuffe Street since the Lord Lieutenant's May Day Ball of 1830. The arrival of the Famine, which convulsed the country between 1845 and 1848, was to coincide with an alteration in the relative prominence of the two hospitals. Due to the forceful character of its founder, St Mark's was to prosper, while more in line with the prevailing abjection, its rival faced a period of temporary eclipse. However, the fact that in these two lay the seed destined for a single blooming, makes each of them part of the extended family and thereby entitled to attention.

Wilde's role as census-taker and statistician made him a formidable keeper of records, something well seen in the annual reports of St Mark's. These appeared regularly from 1845 till amalgamation in 1897 and are our richest single source of information for the late nineteenth century. Through the late 1840s practice was again outstripping premises, and the 1850 report said: 'The Hospital in Mark Street is very incommodious, being quite incapable of containing the crowds, who are obliged to wait on the street.'

In that year the former school of medicine in Park Street, now Lincoln

Place, was acquired by the committee, and the hospital moved to the home it would occupy until amalgamation. Wilde was of course familiar with the building since his student days and aware of its eminent suitability. It is quite clear that the bulk of the purchase money, plus the cost of remodelling the building, totalling nearly £1000, were provided out of his private purse, so that in addition to being the mainspring of the hospital's activities for as long as he lived, he was in every sense the founder.

Though second in time, St Mark's was the larger of the two hospitals which would coalesce in 1897 to form the Royal Victoria Eye and Ear Hospital. Wilde's foundation remains outstanding in the quantity and detail of its archives, which have a unique zest, certainly infused by him. For all of the thirty-two years elapsing between the hospital's first site in Mark Street and the death of Wilde, the force of his personality was strong upon it, nor indeed is it impossible to fancy that the ghost of it still lingers.

3

THE FAMINE AND WHAT FOLLOWED

The historical period in which St Mark's was founded, of itself guarantees reports of particular interest, covering the Famine years and the woeful epidemics that attended them:

> During the season of extreme distress with which the country has been afflicted...some have been received into the Institution, whose state of destitution so far influenced their ophthalmic affections, as to render their admission a matter of urgent necessity. The great amount of epidemic and other sickness during the past year, as well as the immense mortality of the lower classes, has slightly lowered the number of out-patients compared with last year.

This sad extract relates to 1846-47, but worse was to follow, for the next account, published in 1850, tells how in the three years between, the city of Dublin and the country generally had passed through a period of unexampled calamity, producing an increased demand on charities, whose resources had decreased in inverse ratio.

In reflecting the appalling aftermath of the Famine, this commentary also underlines the efforts of some better-off people who tried to mitigate its hardships. Wilde was by now in his prime, and prominent in several walks of life, as surgeon, census commissioner and archaeologist, yet he still gave not only of his time, but also from his pocket, noticed in the generous purchase of the Park Street building. He sought no publicity for this, but the volume of subscriptions to the hospital can be seen as silent recognition of his central role. The personal charity of Irish Quakers was notable. A less successful appeal abroad occasioned a document which in both style and content is so redolent of Wilde as to be considered worthy of reproduction as Appendix B.

The hospital report for 1861 published a remarkable paper read by Wilde in London the previous year. Delivered at the request of the Societé des Bien-Faisances it dealt with the condition of the blind in Ireland. As statistician and eye specialist he showed that since the year 1700 there had been fifteen severe attacks of ophthalmia in the country, roughly one every ten years. Many of them had been associated with potato blight and famine, and coinciding with the arrival of regiments from Egypt a special exacerbation had occurred in 1803.

The first indication of widespread ocular inflammation in the wake of the Great Famine was in 1848 with an outbreak of epidemic ophthalmia among the paupers in Athlone Union Workhouse. The description appals, telling how this 'peculiar influence affected not only the miserable peasantry, suffering from want and exposed to the vicissitudes of weather in their own wretched dwellings' but also 'crowded masses of pauper children in workhouses' as well as regiments of healthy and well-fed soldiers who became affected on visiting the stricken localities. To round up figures cited by Wilde: in a thirteen-year period up to 1861, in the workhouses alone there were 200,000 cases, of whom 500 lost both eyes, 1300 one eye, while 2000 more had visual impairment. The relevance of these figures from 1862 is seen on reaching reports from 1866-71, telling how in February 1867, owing to a severe outbreak of contagious ophthalmia both in dispensary and hospital, it became necessary to discharge all patients who could be safely sent away, and to stop further admissions. The house then underwent a thorough cleansing and repair.

The account goes on to stress how the hospital was under constant pressure to admit patients from all parts of Ireland, referred by the Poor Law guardians, who were by now legally responsible for their maintenance. So briskly did the guardians avail of this right that in the year ending March 1869 the hospital received £369 in payment for Poor Law patients, a very large sum for the period. At times there was such crowding with these patients that the governors were forced to require the Poor Law guardians to furnish with each application a medical certificate stating the nature of the disease, since cases of contagious ophthalmia as found in workhouses could not be admitted with safety alongside other unaffected patients and the limitations of St Mark's did not permit segregation of diseases.

The 1869 report contains a paragraph distilling the knowledge of the time, being simultaneously a treatise on the clinical signs of trachoma, a statement of public health principles and an apologia for the hospital's existence: 'A large number of these pauper patients had been long resident in workhouses, labouring under a very chronic affection of the eyes known as epidemic military or workhouse ophthalmia, attended by granular lids...very easily communicated...spreading rapidly under certain hygienic conditions...endemic when once established, and very difficult to eradicate. It was found impossible to keep the house free from it so long as such patients were admitted; and since treatment of acute diseases, accidents and injuries, as well as restoration or preservation of sight by operation, form the principal objects of the hospital, it has been found necessary, as far as possible, to exclude from the institution patients labouring under this disease. Patients affected with chronic ophthalmia, vascular cornea, and granular lids, will therefore no longer be admitted to the wards, but will be carefully attended to, at the dispensary. There will always be vacancies for the artisans and the deserving poor of Dublin, who have a priority of claim to this charity.'

So effective was this firm and enlightened stand that three years later, in 1872, it was possible to claim that during the previous twelve months the sanitary condition of the establishment had been excellent and that the well-established good repute of the hospital had been confirmed and maintained by the test of the previous year.

In postscript to trachoma's conviction as archvillain in causation of blindness is an 1863 reference to the 'valuable Registry kept at St Mark's Hospital', which was credited by the census commissioners with being a useful agency, especially in the lack of more definite information from official sources. Although this was a case of Wilde the statistician complimenting the hospital of Wilde the oculist, the criticism was valid. Statistics are better now, but the country still lacks a classified State Blind Register.

The epidemic just described was the last thunder roll of the disease which had bedevilled Ireland for so long, although it persisted in endemic form for more than half a century. In 1904 H R Swanzy was to write: 'The inhabitants of Ireland are subject to all the diseases of the eye that are to be found in other countries and to no less degree. But they are more liable than the inhabitants of almost any other land to a severe ophthalmia called trachoma, a terrible disease which is always prevalent, and when neglected commonly leads to complete loss of sight. I believe that, except among Polish Jews and the inhabitants of Finland there are no people so subject to trachoma as our own fellow countrymen.' (With the hindsight of nearly a century we can refute Swanzy's belief, in the knowledge that not race but poor hygienic conditions had formed the predisposing factor.)

J B Story, writing on Sir William Wilde in 1918, gives further insight: 'Trachoma was very prevalent in Ireland during the latter half of the [19th] century.... The disease has greatly decreased since then, although an increase occurred of late years, owing to the immigration of Russian Jews and the strict censorship of the medical officers of American steamship companies, which left crowds of trachomatous individuals stranded in Irish seaports....'

Trachoma lingered on until after World War II, when improved hygiene and housing, together with chemotherapy, accomplished its ultimate extinction in Ireland. Credit for its pursuit during the thirties is due to F J Lavery, who instituted in the RVEEH the energetic regime that helped to stamp it out. Those who were house surgeons fifty years ago will remember the vestigial evidence to be seen in the hospital OPD up to the 1940s. There were the segregated queues of chronic trachoma patients with their distinctive drooping lids, and the hospital 'trachoma tray' bearing drugs and dressings uniquely reserved for their treatment. With the disappearance of these remnants there closed one of the saddest chapters of Irish social history; in effecting this closure, the hospital descending from Wilde and from Swanzy played a definitive role.

From sombre recollection it is a relief to turn to everyday functions of the hospital, which illustrate incidentally the courage and resourcefulness required of a hospital founder. Early accounts of the domestic scene in St Mark's show an appealing frankness, as for instance when dealing with the dietary. In 1857 this was admitted to be 'of the most simple description, such as could be supplied with little risk either of waste or peculation'. For an adult, twenty-four ounces of the best wheaten bread and one quart of the best sweet milk was supplied daily, while on Sundays these quantities were somewhat reduced, the deficit being made up by three half pints of broth, with its meat. Extras, such as tea and sugar, fresh meat and porter, were allowed to some patients, but a corresponding abstraction of the other staples was made. At the time of these allowances (1857) there were twenty beds, and the entire outlay per patient was 1/1d per day. By 1880 the change was phenomenal, the dietary having been still further improved during the previous year and patients getting for dinner a full meat diet of beef or mutton, with vegetables on four days of the week, soup on two days, and bread and gruel on the remaining days.

Down the years the reports reveal little smoulders of resentment against the better-off seeking to gain free treatment. This anger reaches a turgid apotheosis in the report for 1872: 'This system of payment of 6d. per month, adopted at foundation of the institution in 1844 continues to work well, and while the pauper is always attended to gratuitously, those able to afford it pay the trifle cheerfully. Sometimes, either from ignorance or design, persons in good circumstances endeavour to avail of the benefits of the charity, and are no doubt occasionally successful. The officers of the institution are however vigilant and careful to dispense the charity, so far as they can, only to such as are really proper recipients.'

There are revealing glimpses of another world in the early statements of account. Thus for the year ending in March 1846, salaries and nurses' wages totalled £27.16s.6d, while straw came to £1.4s.9d. The latter, used for the patients' beds, was an item so important that a special strawhouse was provided. In the same year leeches cost £19.1s.7d. Leeches were still used regularly up to a hundred years later, just overlapping the penicillin era which consigned them to history.

The index of diseases which proved so helpful to the census commissioner is a feature from the very first report onwards. It has separate sections for conditions of eye and of ear and clearly reflects Wilde's gift for classification. His subdivision of eye cases according to sex and colour of the eyes showed not only his enquiring mind, but also his capacity to adapt: in the course of years he was prepared to drop the classification by colour as the irrelevance that it is, although he continued to the end of his days to regard gender as having pathogenic significance. In general it is seen how he learned by experience, with certain disease entities listed in the earlier reports being quietly dropped in the later ones, strange freakish names like psorophthalmia or aquo-capsulitis, unknown in the canon of today.

The operations recorded were mainly ophthalmic, with a clear majority of cataract extractions. Admissions for squint surgery – which today are teeming – could be as few as in the year 1863 when there were two; this echoed the prevalence of graver illness which had priority. Aural surgery would seem to have been confined to the removal of polypi and foreign bodies and to mastoid operations. The latter procedure constituted a province so dominated by Wilde that the so-called Wilde's Incision, his personal contribution to the technique, has persisted to the present, both as standard surgical practice and as an eponymous tribute to a great innovator.

At St Mark's, rules of behaviour were ordained for patients, porters and nurses. Patients capable of it were to assist in cleaning the hospital, in the washing, and in the pumping of water as directed by the assistant surgeon. Male patients going to the female wards, or vice versa, were subject to instant dismissal. The porter was 'to regulate the dispensary patients on Tuesdays and Fridays: for which he must be able to read and write'. He was to whitewash the privies monthly, to fill the beds with straw and carry them up and down to the wards as often as required. He was also to keep the cistern at the top of the house so full as to command all the water cocks upon the premises. All failures of duty in the foregoing were punishable by fines varying from a penny to a shilling.

When Wilde started his hospital it was yet more than a decade before the name Florence Nightingale would be heard of, still longer before the nursing profession would be born. In St Mark's however he had installed an individual styled the Nurse, and specified her duties. As for the medical attendants, Wilde himself, as well as being autocrat, was for long the sole surgeon in both of the special sense disciplines. From 1845 on there is mention of a shadowy character who was accorded some degree of importance through being listed immediately following the graduate doctors. This was Mr Mapeson, the cupper, who received a small salary and was obliged to attend each dispensary day, and for intern patients whenever required. His primary function was to produce local congestion over a part by applying to it a hollow vessel (the 'cup') from which air had been exhausted to create a vacuum. His other duties are not specified, but from an item of £20 listed for assistant and cupper's salaries, it seems possible that he may sometimes have acted as an unqualified adjutant. The cupper was perhaps paid on piece work, for while his salary in 1864-65 was £18, in a later year it had dropped to £12. The second and last cupper, Mr Winton, doubled in the role of dispenser, but in 1887 he and his calling disappeared from the scene.

The improving role of the resident, possibly a student, is seen in comparing the year of foundation, when there was none, with twenty years later when one of the rooms previously used by the resident assistant had been converted into a ward, and the resident pupil now occupied a room off the boardroom. In 1871 the resident surgeon had a salary of £30; the house surgeon of 1940 received £60 and keep; today's hard-worked incumbent may well be supporting a family.

The list of consultant staff in the early reports reads like a roll-call in a medical Hall of Fame. First there was Wilde himself, from the beginning accompanied by the immortal Robert Graves who was physician to the hospital. His counterpart in surgery was Sir Philip Crampton, Fellow of the Royal Society, a co-founder of Dublin Zoo and four times president of the Royal College of Surgeons in Ireland; he also gained minor fame as describer of the retractor lentis muscle in birds, named Crampton's Muscle in his honour. A celebrated and energetic figure in life, he left instructions that after death his body was to be encased in Roman cement prior to burial in Mount Jerome Cemetery. Crampton was succeeded at St Mark's by William Stokes, whose name lives on in the Stokes-Adams Syndrome known to every medical student from his youth. Even for a large general hospital this team would have been impressive; for a small specialised one it was phenomenal.

Those with a feel for local history and having consciousness of the continuity of things, will recognise in the list of non-medical ancillaries and supporters of St Mark's how there rings an authentic note of nineteenth-century Dublin. From the start, Mr Yeates of Grafton Street was optician to the hospital, while to Hamilton Longs the chemists, thanks was given for a gift of oilsilk, beside acknowledgement of the unusual donation of a leech vase. Both firms are still trading, as are those founded by Alexander Findlater and Sir James Mackey, two early governors of the hospital.

This support of the moneyed merchant class was a feature of St Mark's from the outset. These worthy citizens, together with academics and divines from Trinity College, were the people who steered its fortunes during the nineteenth century, contrasting with today when the State is paymaster and public servants, lawyers and accountants form the backbone of its Council.

While he lived, the prime mover was forever Wilde. There exists no more telling evidence of his ardour than in the Memorial he addressed to the Earl of Eglinton as viceroy in 1858. Presented through Lord Naas, then Secretary for Ireland, this dwelt on the needs of the blind throughout the country, who, entirely unsupported by the State, were indeed in dire plight. As the testament of an individual, it mirrors its author even as he tells his story; as social commentary it reveals a page of Irish history that should not be forgotten. For both reasons it is seen as worthy of inclusion in Appendix C of this volume.

4

ST MARK'S AT ANCHOR

Wilde died in 1876, leaving St Mark's with an established and accepted place in the hearts of his countrymen. An attempt to summarise the height of his achievement would be vanity, but few will disagree that it showed the supreme attribute of flair (defined as 'a selective instinct for what is excellent'). When he died the hospital report came edged in black, in seemly tribute: regardless of famous faults he was a truly great man.

In the years following his death it seemed as if the gods themselves were seeking to demolish St Mark's in a storm of adversity. He was succeeded as senior surgeon by his natural son, Henry Wilson, who had been his assistant for nearly twenty years. Then, in the very report in which Wilson's name stood for the first time as senior, a postscript carried the news of his early death at the age of forty. His portrait shows a grave and well-nourished Victorian gentleman who very likely died of a coronary attack, since we are told that even up to the very day of his fatal illness, his time and skill were always at the disposal of the afflicted poor. His attachment to the hospital was proved in a most practical way: he left it the greater portion of his personal property, although owing to the will being subject to certain life-interests, there was a protracted delay before the bequest became fully effective.

Wilson died within twelve months of his father and in 1877 was in turn

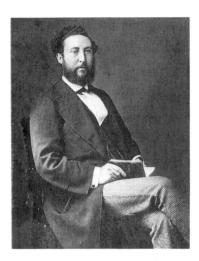

*4.1 Henry Wilson, natural son of Sir William
Wilde. He succeeded his father as surgeon to
St Mark's in 1876 but died after little more
than a year.*

succeeded by the assistant surgeon, Richard Rainsford, whose portrait
shows a handsome young man of romantic appearance. Coming from an
assured background, a Rainsford having been Lord Mayor of Dublin as
early as 1700, his rise to seniority was meteoric, since his first appointment
to St Mark's had been only in 1872 when he was made museum curator, a
period description of pathologist. By the time of Wilde's death he was
listed as 'lecturer in ophthalmic and aural surgery in the Ledwich School of
Medicine' and 'late assistant in Professor Politzer's aural clinique at Vienna'.
Within five years, therefore, he had reached the summit: three years more
and he was gone. We may well guess at his complaint, for we are told that
his period in office was marred by 'frequent and severe attacks of that
malady which eventually carried him off'. The so-called 'portrait
photograph' presented by his mother gives him a look of refined delicacy,
making it no great leap to infer that in then-current phraseology, he
probably died of 'consumption'.

Short though his term of office was, Rainsford was cast in the classic
mould of devoted service; in dedication to the hospital he emulated his
predecessors. Not many weeks before his death he refurbished an entire
ward at his personal expense, being the better able to afford it through
being a bachelor.

The 1880 report was the third in five years to be issued with a

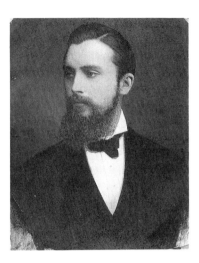

4.2 *Richard Rainsford. He succeeded Henry
Wilson as surgeon to St Mark's in 1877, but
died three years later.*

mourning band on the cover and Rainsford was given a glowing eulogy.
Mrs Rainsford, his mother, remained a hospital subscriber for a number of
years. There is, besides, another item exhaling a faint fragrance after over a
century. This is an acknowledgement of 'Miss ...'s collection for the
Rainsford Ward. (A lady who does not wish her name disclosed.)' The
romantic image is complete.

The report of 1880, his last year in office, was able at long last to
announce the opening of a special ward for contagious ophthalmia,
claiming most gratifying results in treating the disease. For all its optimism
this was but a staging post; the final victory over trachoma was still over
fifty years in the future. The same report enthused over an out-patient
attendance of 11,806 for the past year, giving an average of 31.71
individuals per day. Rainsford was clearly a man of precision born out of
his time; the writer stressed that his figures were no mere estimate, but had
been reached 'with unerring accuracy by a novel and ingenious machine'
which, using numbered dials, counted patients as they passed.

In the history of St Mark's, 1880 was indeed a watershed, separating the
two worlds of ancient and modern. While concrete evidence of this still lay
in the future, it was in 1880 that the Board took heed of a stricture uttered
by the Dublin Hospital Sunday Fund, a financing and overseeing body.
This watchdog in the public interest noted with some asperity the

existence in Dublin of two ophthalmic hospitals doing exactly the same class of work, and suggested a merger might be considered.

Conscientiously the Board sought Counsel's opinion, to be met with the answer that legal articles rendered such an overture outside of its power. With conscience thus quietened, the suggestion fell dormant. Hindsight now tells us that the proposal not only made sense, but was also feasible, albeit with much effort. However, influenced by the legal advice, the will for action froze, and because Counsel's opinion had failed to consider every option, amalgamation was to be deferred for more than a decade.

It is in the person of the senior surgeon appointed in 1880 to succeed Rainsford that we can most surely perceive the bridge between the old and the new. John Benjamin Story first features in the St Mark's report of 1877, when he was resident medical officer. The following year he was made junior surgeon, it being noted that on his election he presented to the hospital the usual donation of £100, which had been invested in India 4% Stock. Two years after, on the death of Rainsford, he found himself senior surgeon, a position he would occupy for almost fifty years. In train with Story was Arthur Benson, who succeeding him as resident medical officer and later as junior surgeon, and who was to remain his close colleague for life.

Reference to 'the usual donation of £100' gives some insight into management arrangements. This is the first noted reference to the practice, which seems to have had a multi-purpose objective, not only in obtaining funds for the hospital but also in securing that a new staff appointee had 'bottom' and would the more certainly identify with his hospital through having a stake in it. There can be no doubt of the Story family's solid support for the hospital, seen in the Rev William Story's donation of one ton of potatoes and in the activities of Mrs Story in collecting for the Artificial Eye Fund. The subject of surgeons' cash involvements with their hospitals will be noted again in connection with the National Eye and Ear Infirmary, which suppressed the practice from the time of Swanzy.

Thus in six years a convulsion shook the St Mark's establishment. The twenty-eighth report, of 1875, noted the staff as comprising Wilde, Wilson and Rainsford; the thirty-third, of 1880, records Story and Benson. There were minor tremors also. We read how in 1878 Miss Molony, the resident lady superintendent appointed the previous year, had since resigned, having defied the Governors' direction to employ a trained nurse acting under her. Her successor Miss Beresford was non-resident; but more tractable, she found no trouble in coping with a trained nurse and efficient staff of assistants. In perusing these reports, there is apparent a marked falling-off both in style and personal warmth from about the time of Rainsford's death onwards. While the yearly details of clinical turnover and classified lists of diseases are meticulous as ever, showing the old zeal unabated, the altered presentation is a reminder that not least of Sir William's gifts was the style that made him a supreme communicator.

Even so, records in the eighties are not wholly lacking items of human and social interest. 'By resolution of the Board the rule has been established allowing each subscriber the privilege of recommending one patient for an artificial eye. Many poor persons, especially domestic servants, having suffered loss of an eye find it difficult afterwards to procure employment unless assisted to replace the absent natural eye by an artificial one. Why this prejudice should exist is difficult to explain; but the fact being so, the necessity for befriending the friendless and homeless dependant becomes all the more urgent.'

The unique Victorian ethic is active in a rare gesture by the Paving Department: '...the space in front of the hospital and thirty feet east and west of same, has been laid with wood pavement by the Corporation, whom the Governors desire to thank for ready acquiescence in a request made in the interest of the sick poor, for whose recovery undisturbed rest is essential.'

Two constant themes in the reports are just as familiar today, the need for funds, and shortage of space for special requirements. A bald statement of conditions comes with: 'The sleeping rooms of the resident staff of nurses and servants are meagre and inadequate, their bedrooms being in the basement which is damp, or in the attic where ventilation is unsatisfactory.' Remedial attempts only compounded the difficulties, since at one stage of renovation, the bathroom was found to be in the way and had to be shifted. It was the only one in the hospital and when sited in the basement had offered hazards to the bathers from the risk of draughts and of the long transit to and from the wards. Pending other arrangements, the bath found a new but scarcely more convenient home in the attic.

Cash statements offer glimpses of problems remote from today. Thus, the travelling expenses of a destitute patient came to £1.5s.0d; flypapers and sundries were 5/7d; and car hire for conveyance of old linen, donation of the Kildare Street Club, amounted to 1/6d. Despite current stringency, today's hospital authority is not constrained to print on its prospectus, in bold type, an announcement to the effect that in all Poor Law applications letters of request must enclose a postal order to cover RETURN TRAVELLING EXPENSES. The penalty for non-compliance with this rule was that such letters would either be left unnoticed or placed at the foot of the waiting list.

The difficulties implicit in the constant struggle imposed by lack of space and lack of funds can be seen as gradually coming to a head. As we approach 1890, the sense of climax looms larger. But first a further strand waits to be woven into the story, and this will form the subject of another chapter.

5

UPS AND DOWNS OF THE NATIONAL

It is time to return to the National Eye and Ear Infirmary, Ryall's foundation of 1814, which was last noticed in 1830 about to enjoy the £600 proceeds of the Lord Lieutenant's Ball. The records tell that soon after this money became available, a house was acquired in Cuffe Street, then a fashionable location, for use as a hospital.

Details of this institution are meagre, although a watercolour exists of the reputed site. The archivist's economy in describing the next few decades almost certainly reflects the dire character of the Famine period and after; moreover, it seems probable that his brevity was that of one writing with insight at the end of an era most people wished to forget. On the Cuffe Street Infirmary, his brief commentary runs: 'It seems to have flourished here, doing much good, until the year 1848, when probably for want of necessary support, impossible to obtain in those times, it languished, although it did not entirely close its doors. On Surgeon Morrison's death, Dr Hildege became surgeon to the Institution.'

Of Surgeon Morrison we know that he graduated MD at Paris in 1822. The first Irish reference to him comes in Watson's *Dublin Almanac* for 1828, where under the heading National Infirmary for Curing Diseases of the Eye, Upper North Gloucester Street, he is mentioned as medical director and operator, his name supplanting Ryall's in this regard. His obituary in the *Directory* for 1858 notes the added qualification of FRCSI and states he was lecturer in ophthalmic surgery, that he practised at 93 Leeson Street and died in January 1857. At the time of his death he had been surgeon to the Cuffe Street Infirmary for twenty-six years. These details permit the inference that Morrison, having been active in Ryall's foundation in Gloucester Street, had continued tenure after its re-establishment in Cuffe Street in 1830.

James Graham Hildege, who succeeded him, was educated at the Carmichael School and at TCD, graduating MRCS, England, in 1852, LK and QCPI in 1853 and FRCSI in 1859. His obituary in the *Medical Press and Circular* states that his practice was altogether ophthalmic and aural. His other appointments included that of surgeon to the North City Eye Dispensary and lecturer on ophthalmic surgery to the Carmichael School.

The early years of his tenure at Cuffe Street are obscure, but from 1866 on, bound hospital records are fortunately available. The silence between 1830 and 1866 is regrettable, but the archivist editing the renewed records stoutly insists that the tradition was unbroken from 1814. The link was probably a slender one since we know that from lack of funds there were no admissions for some years prior to 1862. No one can doubt that this situation was a further reflection of the immense catastrophe the nation had undergone.

However, by 1865 there were two wards, and that year saw the performance of thirty-four operations, including sixteen cataracts. In addition, the scope of the hospital was widened to include diseases of women and children. 'Having been for a long period an Institution solely for diseases of the eye and ear, some years since it was considered that its sphere of usefulness would be greatly increased by the addition of a dispensary for the diseases of women and children; not for the mere paupers, but for those who could afford a small – and only a small – fee, the wives of mechanics and artisans.' While this fresh activity indicated welcome renascent energy after the Famine, in the context of a hospital for the special senses it showed a confused sense of classification, as if the Committee had somehow lost direction. However, the National's renaissance was soon to come; its champion was in waiting.

Besides J G Hildege as ophthalmic and aural surgeon, the staff at this time comprised William Colles and William Burke as general surgeon and physician respectively, both being also attached to Dr Steevens' Hospital. Also a familiar figure recurs in the person of Mr Winton, who as cupper is the only individual recorded as holding the unique distinction of working for this hospital and Wilde's simultaneously.

Hildege remained surgeon until his death in 1870. His stay in office invites little comment beyond that offered by C E Fitzgerald who, in writing of the period, said that during it the Eye and Ear Department of the hospital was at a very low ebb, owing to neglect stemming from Dr Hildege's ill-health for some time prior to his death. Despite this poor health, in the last year of his life Hildege became secretary of the committee of management, a role to be made significant by his successor. In lamenting his passage the reporter remarked that less than forty-eight hours before his death he had operated for cataract on a woman who 'now rejoices in perfect vision and would fain be able to thank him'.

Unawares, in 1870 Irish ophthalmology had reached a point of climax. Sir William Wilde would be active in the flourishing St Mark's for another six years; in succession to Hildege at the 'National' a new star was in the ascendant, one destined to shine on coming decades as clearly as Wilde had illumined his. The separate traditions they represented were irresistibly converging, although a further quarter century was to pass before they would coincide.

The new surgeon in Cuffe Street was Dr Henry Rosborough Swanzy, who had graduated from Trinity in 1865, the son of a Dublin solicitor who was a Freeman of the city. The family derived recently from County Monaghan and more remotely from a military ancestor who came to Ireland in the Williamite train. The second name, Rosborough, related him to a family of linen drapers, also from the north of Ireland, whose Dublin representative had been that same Samuel who with ten others founded the Sick and Indigent Roomkeepers' Society in the city in 1790. It has not been possible to establish this individual's relationship to Henry Swanzy but, as Samuel died in 1832, his kinship to the child born in 1844 seems probable. This is genetically the more likely since the work of the Society, now Dublin's oldest charity and a splendid example of non-sectarian philanthropy, has strong humanitarian reverberations in the lifework of Henry Swanzy.

Like Wilde, on qualifying Swanzy had sought continental Europe for specialised studies, identifying Germany and Austria as the well-springs of ophthalmic knowledge. He went at a time momentous for his chosen discipline. German-speaking Europe was then studded with names destined for inscription in the ophthalmological canon. It was there he learned to be familiar not only with the science itself but with many of the formulators of basic concepts in an emerging specialty.

It was the year of the Austro-Prussian War. Arriving in time for the campaign of 1866, he served in a non-combatant role as a surgeon with

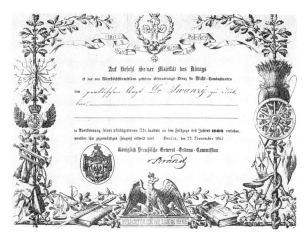

5.1 *Certificate accompanying the Commemorative Cross for Non-Combatants, bestowed in November 1867 on 'Dr Swanzy of Dublin in recognition of his loyal participation'. It was issued on behalf of the King of Prussia by the Royal Prussian General Orders Commission.*

the Prussian army, seeing action at the battle of Sadowa. Field service ended, and he studied at both Vienna and Berlin. In the latter he became assistant for three years in the private clinic of Professor Albrecht von Graefe, a name revered as the founder of scientific ophthalmic surgery. During these journeyman years, Swanzy became a fluent German speaker; still extant in the writer's possession are notebooks from the time spent with von Graefe, in which the observations oscillate from English to German and back again with bilingual ease.

Finally equipped with the skills he sought, he returned to Ireland in 1870, where in the following year he succeeded Hildege at the National Eye and Ear Infirmary; he was also made consultant to the Adelaide Hospital. This last connection deserves somewhat particular mention, since with a brief intermission it lasted until he died and underlined facets of his own character and philosophy. While it did not offer the teaching opportunity he required, his loyal attachment to it reflected the attraction of like to like, through the sharing of a common ethos. As a Protestant hospital dedicated to Crown and Establishment, the Adelaide epitomised the constants of his own philosophy. Nevertheless, for Swanzy this philosophy did not inhibit a broadness of outlook which today might pass as ecumenical; it certainly guided his own sure instinct that sectarian trends in a special sense hospital serving the whole community must be avoided.

By an odd coincidence, Swanzy's ultimate foundation came to be sited

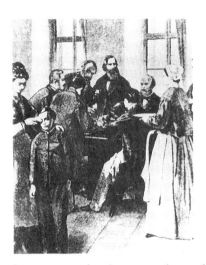

5.2 *Scene from von Graefe's clinic in Berlin, 1867-69. The sketch shows, centre, von Graefe operating; to the right of the picture Dr Swanzy, seated, is administering the anaesthetic, and to the left a boy with eye padded is being led away.*

in Adelaide Road, the connection of name being entirely fortuitous. Despite the element of chance the similarity was enough to perplex the public imagination. To the present day the existence of an Adelaide Hospital in Peter Street and of an Eye and Ear Hospital in Adelaide Road leads to regular public confusion as to their identities. The shade of Swanzy can permit a smile at the association.

The impact of his arrival at the National was almost instant, but clearly he wrought change by consent and not duress. The first thing to be arranged was a change of address from Cuffe Street where 'the sanitary arrangements had become intolerable'. Accordingly in May 1872 the infirmary was moved to 97 St Stephen's Green, where with new premises, the new era in management was soon manifest. A significant feature of Swanzy's appointment was that he was not only surgeon to the hospital but also secretary of the committee of management, as the ailing Hildege was before him. This put him at the heart of affairs, imparting a power he wielded wisely and never relinquished.

No better assessment of his character exists than that sketched in the *Lancet* after he died: 'Swanzy's personal character was as rare as his scientific attainments. Intelligence, quickness of perception, judgment, struck even the casual observer. But to those who knew him the prevailing characteristic was his singlemindedness. Whatever his objective was – the treatment of a patient, the success of his hospital, the prosperity of the College – he devoted himself to it without permitting anything to turn him aside.'

Prior to 1873, details of the hospital's management structure are uncertain, but a firm basis existed from that year on when for the first time a committee of management was established. On its formation the members' first business was to declare themselves unwilling to act unless all private ownership in the institution was resigned into their hands, a condition that had the full concurrence of the medical members, Dr Kirkpatrick the physician and Dr Swanzy the surgeon. The inference that, ex officio, both had some personal stake in the foundation is confirmed in the continuing minute: 'The Committee however considered it right to indemnify these gentlemen in the amount at which their respective shares had been valued between themselves.' As it was considered inadmissible to use any of the charitable funds of the infirmary for such purpose, a special subscription list was opened enabling the appropriate adjustment to be made. The result was to ensure that all future appointments to the medical staff would rest entirely with the committee and that nepotism would be obviated.

This stroke in other words saw the birth of a voluntary hospital. While no details of the previous arrangement have survived it would appear that certain members of the medical staff had, vested in their persons, the title to some part of the hospital possessions. Swanzy's clear mind saw this for the quagmire it was, and this early deed was a necessary clearing of the ground he was about to occupy. The arrangement he demolished may have been analogous to what still prevailed in St Mark's five years later, when Dr Story on appointment presented the 'usual donation of £100' which finished up in India 4% Stock.

Viewed in perspective, Swanzy's prescience in causing the National to put its house in order was admirable, a prudent act of preparation by a young man still on the threshold. His years in Germany had taught him more than surgery and his flair for administration inevitably owes something to them. The incident offers a lesson illustrating how, even over a century ago, the principle of impartiality in conduct of a public body was recognised as essential. As a further axiom the specific outlawing of nepotism shows that human nature has not altered.

However lest it be thought there was any scope for private gain in the running of the institution, it is necessary only to note the constant pleas for financial support in the years after the start of management by committee. For instance, during the last quarter of 1876, when funds were so depleted it became incumbent to refuse any but the most urgent cases, it is recorded that 'rather than permit some anxious and distressing cases to go unalleviated, the medical officers personally bore the expense attendant on admission'.

If the records of the National are less flamboyant than those of St Mark's, they always contain a strongly practical element that is sometimes even prophetic. 'It is a matter of note that while so much is done for the support of the blind (or of those who have been let go blind), so little is done for those who are going blind.' So did this small hospital perceptively anticipate the prophylactic role of community care today.

From a committee originating in the prosperous professional and business classes, real concern for social conditions of the time is evident in the entry: 'The work of this hospital is most useful and important; for in the case of a poor man blindness entails misery not only on himself, but on his whole family: while even minor maladies of the eyes involve temporary loss of employment or permanent diminution of bread winning power.' Contributions to the hospital mirror the rise of modern industrial society, the subscribers including many employers whose names live on, such as Guinness, Jacob and Arnott, while John Jameson is even a member of the committee.

Apart from dearth of funds, the next most constant plea concerned the need for expansion. In 1873, soon after Swanzy's accession, the infirmary, questing for improvement, had established a dispensary for diseases of the throat. The first of its kind in Dublin, this was something marrying better with eye and ear than did diseases of women and children, which before long ceased to be a concern of the infirmary. In announcing the throat dispensary, allusion was made to the benefit in treatment of such diseases afforded by the newly invented laryngoscope. With this expanded activity, space problems persisted, and in 1878, due to bed shortage, the committee reluctantly gave up the private ward, placing three new beds in it.

The movement to Molesworth Street was a great improvement, and the number of beds was doubled. At the new premises an out-patients department was specially built, whose entrance by Frederick Lane, now Setanta Place, followed in Wilde's earliest footsteps and secured for this humble thoroughfare a second citation in Irish ophthalmological history. This OPD had separate waiting rooms for men and women, with an ample consulting room for eye diseases and distinct rooms for ear ailments.

The attention to detail seen in the records gives a sharp image of Swanzy the man. Nothing but the best would do. Even in the confined premises at Stephen's Green, with a mere dozen or so beds, a new operating couch had been procured from Heidelberg which, carriage included, cost £15.5s.3d. 'The new couch is of that kind most highly approved on the Continent and in America.' To a great extent, plans for the Molesworth Street hospital were based on London models. There were twenty-four beds with a separate out-patient department; a central-heating system profiting both interns and externs represented quite advanced technology for the early 1880s. Other thoughtful arrangements included such details as a food lift, a bathroom and provision for a fire hose, while in 1886 redecoration by the then sophisticated method of oil-painting made the OPD 'the most perfect dispensary in the city'.

As with Wilde and St Mark's the reports in themselves reflected the persona of their author. The one from Cuffe Street had come in a plain cover, but on moving to St Stephen's Green this was replaced with a picture of No 97, the hospital's name being blazoned with the foundation date, AD 1814. It carried a quotation from Goethe: 'Sterben ist nichts – doch leben und nicht sehen, Das ist ein Unglück'. (To die matters not, but to live yet not see – that is misfortune.) With the transfer to Molesworth Street this motto remained, but it was now accompanied by a tasteful line-drawing of Tobias and the Angel in the curing of Tobit's blindness.

From the first moment of his appointment to the National, Swanzy's boundless ambition for it certainly envisaged a teaching role for its staff, then comprising himself and Fitzgerald. They had arrived in 1871, and despite the mountain of reorganisation that faced them, by 1873 Fitzgerald was noted as being also ophthalmic surgeon to the Richmond Hospital and lecturer in the subject at the associated Carmichael School of Medicine. Meantime Swanzy, lifelong oculist to the Adelaide Hospital, is seen by 1876 to have become lecturer to Dr Steevens' Hospital School of Medicine (the Adelaide having no formal teaching centre based on it). In 1877 he became professor of ophthalmic and aural surgery at the College of Surgeons in succession to Henry Wilson. Later still he was to be examiner to the Royal University. In the course of time his increasing involvement with a wider world saw him dropping all extraneous appointments except the Adelaide, and limiting clinical teaching to the National Eye Infirmary, epicentre of his actions.

As time slips by and 1890 approaches, the records show the first printed reference to the possibility of amalgamation with St Mark's. To those with insight there are other signs: in 1883 the appointment of P W Maxwell as assistant surgeon, and of Louis Werner as clinical assistant in 1886. Rather than mere names added to a list; these people were the start of a legend; down the coming decades, through their children and

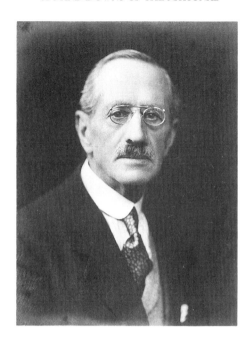

*5.3 Louis Werner Senior (above) and Louis Werner
Junior (below) were between them associated with
the Eye and Ear Hospital and its predecessor, St
Mark's, for over a hundred years.*

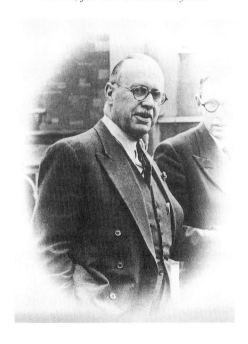

successors, they were to cast a long shadow on Irish ophthalmology deep into the twentieth century.

The National's constant shortage of both beds and money reached a climax when the report of 1890 announced that rather than continued talk about enlargement, a possible union with St Mark's was being seen as a better option. The moment of truth had arrived and been acknowledged. The report proceeded: 'This union has for many years been advocated by the Committee of Management of this hospital, wherefore earlier this year it was with pleasure they received an invitation from the Board of St Mark's to consider with them the feasibility of the project.'

This, if not a *volte-face,* was a deviation from the traditional *laissez-faire* attitude of the hospitals. It has been shown how St Mark's had tentatively explored the possibility of a merger some ten years previously, but deterred by the adverse opinion of learned Counsel, had shelved the question indefinitely. The National, as the smaller unit, had been slow to pursue an idea which, if realised, would extinguish its independent existence and might suppress its identity. Given two such stances, convergence of the parties was possible only with intervention from outside. The origin and result of this mediation forms the next part of the story.

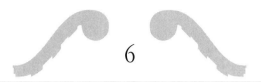

6

A MARRIAGE OF UNLIKE MINDS

In 1890 the anomaly presented by a city with two specialised hospitals, providing identical services and lying within a quarter of a mile of one another, at last became subject to public commentary. Under the arrangements of the day several visiting committees were charged with supervising management of hospitals and similar institutions. These were the City Hospitals Committee of Dublin Corporation, the Visiting Committee of the Dublin Hospital Sunday Fund, a private charity, and a Government Board for Superintendence of the Dublin Hospitals. Their visits were dreaded occasions for managing authorities since upon them depended the payment of certain running costs; also because the inspectors were wont to arrive without warning.

On this occasion confabulation between the inspecting bodies was obvious, manifested in marked unanimity of opinion on the part of all three. Ever a model of lucidity, St Mark's Hospital report for 1889-90 tabulated conclusions reached by the three separate visitations of the year gone by. They showed a common denominator. In findings given independently, but all based on grounds of economy and efficiency, each committee would favour amalgamation of the two hospitals into one large institution.

The response by the two Boards was immediate and orderly. Within two months a joint committee comprising four representatives from each hospital had not merely convened, but after five meetings had delivered its final report, with findings so important as to merit quotation at some length:

> We have come to the conclusion that one large united Hospital would be in all respects better than the two existing institutions.
>
> The proposed United Hospital should contain 120 beds, as the two existing hospitals contain nearly 80, and are both constantly refusing applicants for want of space.
>
> The new Out-patient Department must contain space for double the number of out-patients that can at present be accommodated at either institution at a given time.
>
> To obtain the additional beds and extra space in the Out-patient Department, it would be necessary to build what would practically be a new hospital.
>
> In conclusion, your joint committee earnestly urge their respective boards not to allow the present opportunity of uniting the hospitals to drop, from a difficulty in collecting funds; more especially as they fully believe that such a union will become more difficult in the future.

Henceforward the aim of a United Hospital was to be viewed as Dublin's destiny. That destiny was still seven years in the future, an interval during which the painfully slow convergence was diligently charted in the still separate annual reports of the hospitals. However, these printed reports lack the urgency dwelling in the month-to-month Council minutes of the National, records fortunately still available to convey a sense of how it was to be in the front line during this long encounter. While couched in the third person, these notes record Swanzy's insights and effectively comprise a diary of the period.

First came an all-important Counsel's opinion. Delivered by Serjeant Jellett, QC, and traversing the ground covered ten years before, it took in options not then considered. It stated that the Court of Chancery lacked the power to effect amalgamation, which would require an Act of Parliament, but that if the latter were to be promoted by Government there would be little expense to the petitioners.

Though the National was roughly half the size of St Mark's, its board made clear from the start that it saw the discussion as one between equals, and by going politely on the offensive it secured early vantage points from which it never retreated. Pointing out that Wilde's Deed of Trust appeared to interdict a union with any other institution, it pressed St Mark's Board to clarify its position both as to this, and – should amalgamation progress – as to whether the Lincoln Place site would be a bargaining factor. A long letter on these and other issues was signed by Swanzy as honorary secretary to the National, but little insight is needed to see him acting the clever role of the board's mouthpiece when in fact he was chief formulator of its policies.

Throughout Swanzy's career at the National, he had enjoyed the staunch support of his colleague, C E Fitzgerald, a colourful personality in his own right. A competent doctor, he was also an art connoisseur, and because of this second interest, being as it were in possession of a dual mandate, he was never as single-minded as Swanzy in his dedication to hospital affairs. The senior surgeon at St Mark's by this time was J B Story, a figure of worth and integrity indeed, but on the evidence, not one to resist the administrative dynamism of a Swanzy. Next to him stood Arthur Benson, who despite achievements meriting a high relief bronze memorial in the hospital and the eponymous honour of having a disease named for him in the textbooks, somehow fails to emerge three-dimensionally from the archives.

Thus of the four ranking surgeons at the time when amalgamation was proposed, Swanzy stood paramount in possessing not only a full grasp of the situation but also the competence and will to achieve it. Of course there was also input by various important lay figures, Board members prominent in civic and legal circles who gave weighty service in realising what was the dream of them all. Yet not belittling their efforts, in the last analysis it is mere recognition of fact to discern Swanzy at the heart of every endeavour in bringing that dream to reality.

Most of 1891 was occupied in establishing a legal format for the proposed amalgamation, and considering whether the bill to introduce it should be Government-sponsored or private. The final decision was for the latter. While the National's Board remained its nominal negotiator, Swanzy was the grey eminence behind all initiatives; he seldom took direct action, except for one approach to the attorney general, already a known partisan. St Mark's main contribution to the joint effort was the legal one of setting its own house in order, and of endorsing and amending the several drafts of agreement between the two sides.

By January 1893, a finally amended agreement had been received from the Board of St Mark's and assented to by the National, with the seemingly innocuous rider that 'the committee did not like the name proposed by the St Mark's board for the proposed new hospital, viz. "St Mark's and National

Eye and Ear Hospital" '. Accordingly the honorary secretary was authorised to confer with the authorities at St Mark's and endeavour to obtain their consent to change the name to 'The Dublin Eye and Ear Hospital' or 'The Royal Dublin Eye and Ear Hospital'.

From such small beginnings arose a conflict which was to sour relations between the two bodies for far longer than was warranted. Many wars are fought for petty causes and this was no exception, the sticking point on each side being a praiseworthy reverence for historical origins. It is astonishing that the battle lines defined as a result of this simple issue remained largely unaltered from January 1893 until the end of May 1894. As perceived by St Mark's, the point of contention hinged on a joint Governors' meeting of 4 December 1892 when it was claimed a decision had been made to adopt the name 'St Mark's and National Eye and Ear Hospital'. For its part the Board of the National was convinced that this name threatened quickly to obliterate all memory of their smaller hospital, since it was so liable to acquire the abbreviation of simply 'St Mark's'. Furthermore, the National queried whether any minutes had been taken at the meeting in question, and embarrassingly St Mark's proved unable to confirm that they had, the alleged minute having been compiled retrospectively from notes taken by 'a gentleman' who had happened to substitute for the secretary in the latter's absence.

As the Governors of Wilde's foundation continued to insist that the name of St Mark's should be incorporated in the new title, being 'already surrounded with associations which they prize and which they think should not lightly be allowed to die', so did the committee of the National write to say that they regretted the name proposed should be almost the only name they would object to, just as they were aware the St Mark's Board would prefer it to any other. Holding no strong views on a compromise name, they suggested the Dublin Ophthalmic Hospital or suchlike as being suitable, and submitted a sample letterhead on which this name was subtitled with those of the constituent hospitals.

While from its own viewpoint each hospital saw its argument as an absolute, neither was so blinded as to attempt reneging on the intent to unite. In the first quarter of 1893, there passed between managements an exchange of letters in which a display of sweet reason by each sought to allay a still fixed determination on the part of the other. During this exchange, signature of the agreement between the two lay in suspense, even though it was already so far advanced that the proposed signatories for the National had been nominated, one of them incidentally that John Jameson whose name was destined for celebrity elsewhere.

By May of 1893 the situation had all but frozen. Letters had become stiffer and more formal, and this chilly politeness was the prelude to a period of about six months during which the two parties nursed their wounded pride and literally sulked. All correspondence ceased and a stony silence in the minutes is more eloquent than words.

Unseasonably, the thaw started in December. In that month a letter from the National to St Mark's sought the latter's consent to the appointment of an arbitrator on the vexed question of a name for the new institution. It further suggested there should be no difficulty in finding some impartial person, who, not being a subscriber to the funds of either hospital, would be acceptable to both parties. The Master of the Rolls was mentioned as a possibility in this capacity if he should agree.

However, after the long cold silence this placatory overture was hardly likely to go uncontested. While agreeing in principle, the Board of St Mark's considered the proposal to be premature until Governors of the National would have signed the draft Bill. It also suggested variation of the arbitration mechanism by the setting up of a Board comprising one representative from each hospital, under the chairmanship of Dr Ingram, the president of the Royal Irish Academy.

At least the parties had now come to grips and with care the delicate trading could proceed. Predictably after such a bout, both sides were touchy. In accepting Dr Ingram's name as broker the National thought it better to have him as sole arbitrator, allowing each hospital several representatives to argue the respective cases. St Mark's assented to the first premise but preferred that the arbitrator should have no more than two advisers, one from each side; steadfast in choice, it opted for the originally disputed title in its long form.

The National's response was a trenchant refusal to have the case submitted 'in the form proposed by your Board, as they have never and will not now contend for any particular name, merely that it should be one which will not give undue prominence to either of the present institutions, such as, for example a name already submitted by my Committee, viz. "The Dublin Ophthalmic Hospital, being an amalgamation of St Mark's Ophthalmic Hospital founded AD 1844 by Sir William Wilde, and the National Eye and Ear Infirmary, founded 1814 by Surgeon Ryall", – or some other neutral name; and the Committee cannot see any objection to leaving a discretionary power in the hands of the Arbitrator.'

The arguments continued in futile multiplication until at last it seems to have dawned on these serious-minded adults that their behaviour was generating only mutual frustration of a common objective. So it remained until quite suddenly in June 1894 came the long-awaited reconciliation and at last the lion lay down with the lamb. The exact sequence of events leading to this near-miracle is not traceable through the pages of the minute book; the explanation may well be of an internecine feud being finally settled by sensible men sitting together across a table. Time has proved how well the breach has healed. The arbitration itself was completed in a few weeks and Dr Ingram wrote that after careful consideration of all the facts and arguments his award was that the amalgamated institution be called the Dublin Eye and Ear Hospital etc (going on to define the formative units, exactly in the terms furnished by the National). The decision was noted and accepted without comment.

The fact that there was no triumphalism, which would have been improper and disruptive, can after nearly a century be fairly ascribed to Swanzy, whose quality of singlemindedness is nowhere better seen than in this incident. Both parties had lost titles dear to them, but in the light of an important new entity having been created it was his nature to look constructively to the future. Looking back from our time, the pity is that the awarded title was not retained, give or take a royal prefix. For apart from the fact that Royal Victoria institutions spread like a rash at the time of the Queen's Jubilee, it is true that Victoria no more loved Ireland than Ireland loved her. It remains Ireland's loss that the name of her capital city does not, as intended, adorn what is in every sense a capital hospital.

Pl 1 The Royal Victoria Eye and Ear Hospital, 1992.

Pl 2 St Mary's Hospital and Dublin's Eye Infirmary, situated at No 36 Lower Ormond Quay from 1819 to 1831.

Pl 3 Dublin Infirmary for Diseases of the Eye and Ear (1872–75), situated at No 23 Ely Place.

Pl 4 First site of St Mark's Ophthalmic Hospital for Diseases of the Eye and Ear (then called the Dispensary for Diseases of the Eye and Ear), located from 1841 to 1844 in Frederick Lane at the rear of No 11 Molesworth Street.

Pl 5 Site in Mark Street adjoining St Mark's Parish Church from which Wilde's hospital derived its dedication. His previous venture in South Frederick Lane had been designated the Eye and Ear Dispensary.

Pl 6 Building at Park Street (1850–1904), now Lincoln Place, the third and final site before amalgamation of St Mark's Ophthalmic Hospital for Diseases of the Eye and Ear. Inset: the original building before enlargement in 1862.

Pl 7 Early sites of the National Infirmary for Diseases of the Eye.
a) No 5 North Cumberland Street (1817–28).
b) Upper Gloucester Street (1828–29).
c) No 10 Cuffe Street (1830–46). It later moved to No 12, and transferred to No 97 St Stephen's Green in 1872.

Pl 8 Seventh and penultimate site of the National Eye and Ear Infirmary (1873–1880) at No 97 St Stephen's Green.

Pl 9 Eighth and final site before amalgamation of the National Eye and Ear Infirmary, from 1880 to 1904, at No 13 Molesworth Street.

1

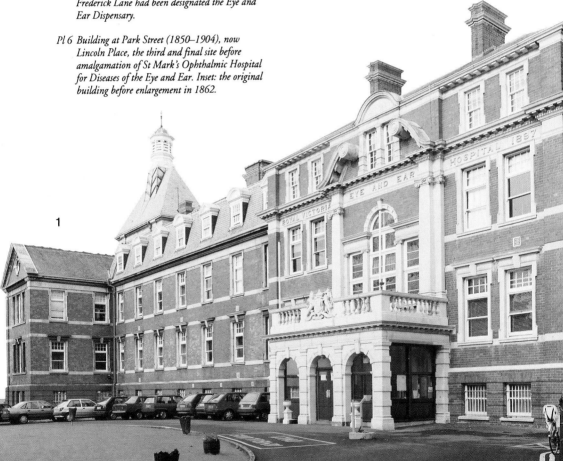

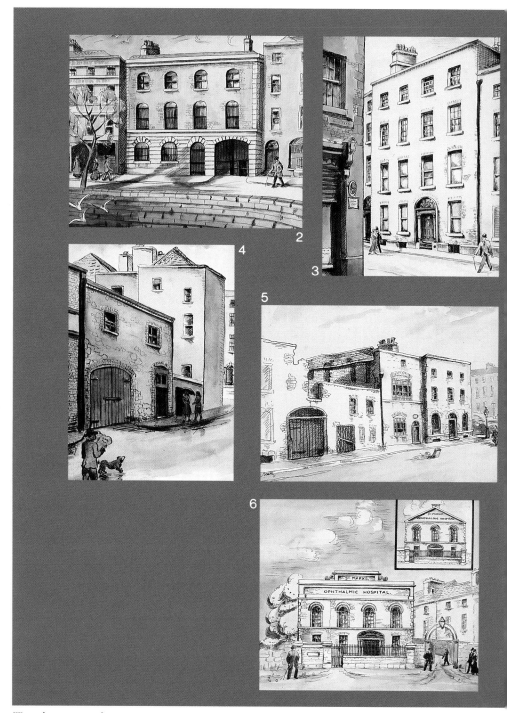

Watercolour paintings of various nineteenth-century eye hospitals in Dublin, presented to the Royal Victoria Eye and Ear Hospital throu

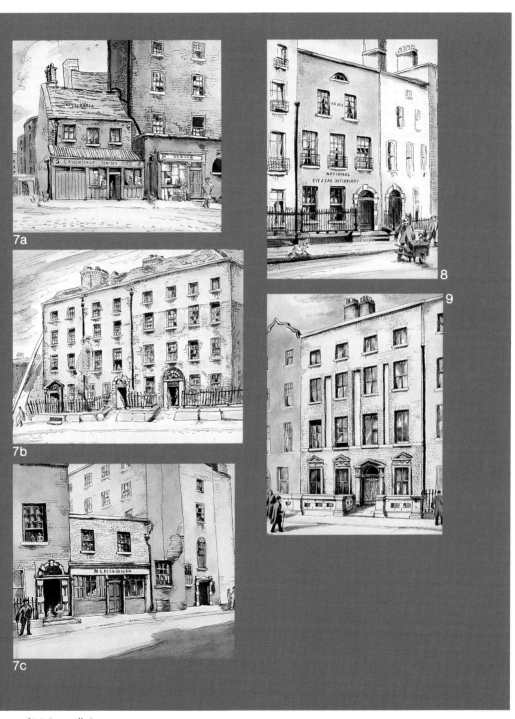

7a

7b

7c

8

9

rosity of L B Somerville-Large.

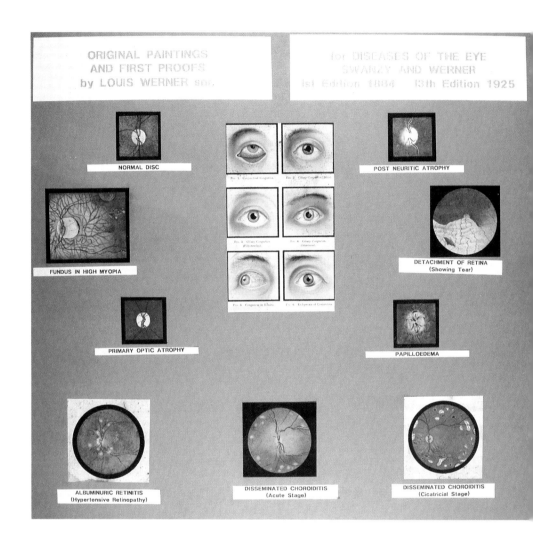

Pl 10 Original ophthalmic paintings executed by Louis Werner Senior, to illustrate later editions of Diseases of the Eye *(Swanzy and Werner). First published in 1884, the textbook's thirteenth and last edition appeared in 1925. The paintings were presented to the Eye and Ear Research Foundation by Louis Werner Junior. They are here represented in colour through his generosity and that of his widow Mrs Patricia Werner.*

7

HOMELESS AND BEGGING

It was not until January 1895 that signature of the Deed of Amalgamation by both hospital Boards could be reported; within weeks a new body, the Joint Amalgamation Committee, came into existence. Appropriately, first mention of this arose in the context of funding, a matter of major importance to the new venture.The agreement between the two hospitals stipulated that £10,000 towards building should be collected prior to petitioning Parliament for the enabling legislation. Good husbandry and the generosity of legators helped towards amassing this amount, but much the greatest increment came in May 1896 through staging a monster bazaar in the RDS grounds. At that period the bazaar was a universally used means of fund-raising, part of the trick being to hit on a name that would catch the public imagination.

Real examples of such events are mentioned in stories by James Joyce, the Araby for instance in *Dubliners,* and in *Ulysses* the Mirus which raised £4000 for a new operating theatre in Jervis Street Hospital. The present occasion became memorable on two counts. Firstly, by the outrageous but brilliant pun of naming the bazaar 'Cyclopia' (its objective being the securing of One Eye Hospital) it gained the publicity desired by all fund-raising, incidentally becoming a legend that lasted in folk memory for decades. Secondly, by collecting £7,000 towards the targetted £10,000 it brought so much nearer the next step to realising physical unity in a new building.

The sum of £10,000 was no magic figure, calculated to resolve all difficulties. It was indeed just an aiming target, specified in the Act as a figure to be accumulated in evidence that the parties were in earnest; until this sum was reached the assets of the existing hospitals would not be made available to the new institution. The final goal was to be something like today's concept of the Universe, always receding, forever unattainable. Hence when the nominated amount was realised by January 1897 the need for future efforts by this new generation of founders was only spurred. They faced a formidable task since besides enlargement of the site or acquisition of a new one the planned expansion envisioned a fifty per cent increase of joint bed-capacity. But now, at least the die was cast, and the only path lay forward.

When at the beginning of 1897 the petition requesting enabling legislation was signed, it found itself accorded a Government response so prompt that within months the new hospital was incorporated by Act of Parliament. The idea of substituting 'Royal Victoria' for 'Dublin' in the hospital's definitive title was moved in a formal motion laid before the Board of the National. Proposed by Perrin the honorary treasurer, with Swanzy as seconder, the motion was adopted without objection from either hospital, and granted royal approval later in the year.

In July 1897 the first Council meeting of the new hospital convened, in circumstances exceptional if not unique. Two long-standing institutions had been dissolved, yet continued to function. A new one had been created, yet had no physical presence save in the separate premises of the predecessors it had supplanted. On the members of Council, derived equally from two constituencies, fell the task of evolving a new corporate identity which, had they known it, would not take physical shape for another seven years. As a single head they would govern a new-born monstrosity with two bodies. Despite such complexities this Council, by reason of a major decision taken at the outset of its existence, effectively vindicated itself for posterity. At its first meeting on 15 July 1897, at which the appointment of honorary officers was the main business, Henry R Swanzy was unanimously elected honorary secretary, a position he was to hold to the end of his days. This decision was to be of definitive significance in the success of the new venture.

While appointment of its honorary officers was a natural priority for a newly established Council, the alacrity of Swanzy's election to this responsible post was a measure of the esteem his administrative ability

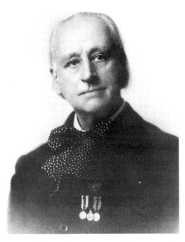

7.1 *C E Fitzgerald, oculist extraordinary, who crowned a unique career by becoming president of the Royal College of Physicians in Ireland.*

commanded. It was unusual for a hospital Board, consisting largely of laymen, to nominate a practising doctor to such a position of power in his own place of practice. However, having proved himself at the National, the quality of that achievement would have clinched this further selection. Such an appointment would be almost unimaginable today; its success on this occasion was based on Swanzy's rock-like integrity. His track record now was such as to win confidence not only from lay members and his long-time colleagues at the National, but also from his newer associates at St Mark's. From now on, the decisive voice was to be always his, and his the opinion ever sought, on topics that ranged from cost of patients' diets to phrasing a letter to the Home Secretary, from the suitability of a site to choice of porter's uniform.

Initially, his medical associates on Council were three, namely C E Fitzgerald, colleague and friend for many years at the National, together with John B Story and Arthur Benson from St Mark's. Within months of the new hospital being launched, Fitzgerald resigned, an event foreshadowed in the founding articles which specified that the initial four medical members of Council should drop to three at occurrence of the first vacancy and so remain thereafter. The pre-arranged resignation enabled the courteous Fitzgerald to concentrate on other interests. He had deferred it for two reasons, being wishful to complete twenty-five years service, and through concern that his juniors would not be overridden in the transition.

His letter of resignation acknowledged a long and cordial association with Swanzy.

Fitzgerald was also an art connoisseur and he thenceforth gave more time to this interest. He did not abandon medical practice however and years later he became president of the Royal College of Physicians of Ireland, to which he presented the presidential badge still in use. His name will be recognised by some as the donor of several important pictures in the National Gallery of Ireland, which carry an acknowledgement to him. When Swanzy died, he wrote a moving obituary, constituting an important biographical source for our knowledge of its subject.

Other manoeuvres for setting the new institution on a firm base were still pending. Chief among them was a need to find a distinguished president of Council, a dignitary whose eminence would impart prestige to the public face of the hospital. First choice fell on Lord Iveagh, who courteously acknowledged but declined the honour, as he had long since made it a rule not to accept any office unless he could accord it sufficient time. Lord Holmpatrick likewise declined, and the lot fell finally on Viscount Monck, a gentleman who in accepting the distinction was guileless enough to admit that he had not even been aware of the amalgamation. He made amends by serving the hospital long and diligently, remaining president until his resignation in 1919.

The great concern of all now was to further the realisation of a new building. A saga with many sub-plots, this topic offers a chapter in itself and will so be treated. Meanwhile, in the now united institutions, the wonted work went on, as it were under the slogan: 'Business as usual – under new management.' The registrars of both previous hospitals were discharged with three months notice. A single successor, sought by advertisement, was chosen from 104 applicants. He was to have a salary of £100 a year, plus commission on subscriptions, the percentage being doubled if they were secured by his own efforts. The successful applicant was Edward Parker, whose industry is abundantly evident in the handwritten letter books still available. His choice was no accident. As secretary to the National for the past decade, he was obviously known to and approved by Swanzy.

Much effort was exercised in procurement of an official seal for the hospital. A design committee was composed of Swanzy and Fitzgerald, the latter a natural choice because of his artistic bent. The selected entry, by a Mr Bell, was awarded a premium of five guineas. Executed by Waterlows of London, the seal shows the seated figure of a woman protectively shielding two kneeling forms. At ground level the disappearing shape of a

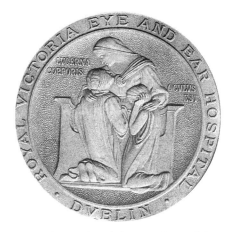

7.2 *The hospital seal shows a classical figure in protective pose, and carries a Latin motto: 'The eye is the lantern of the body.'*

serpent is doubly allusive: in itself the creature sacred to Aesculapius, mythical god of healing, it is therefore symbolic of the healing art; the act of disappearance refers to banishment of evil, here meaning disease. Investing the tableau is the motto, taken from Matthew vi.22: Lucerna Corporis Oculus Est, the Eye is the Lantern of the Body. The actual seal was treated with an almost sacred reverence, each use of it being recorded in Council minutes, while the keys securing it were in the keeping of the two senior surgeons, Swanzy and Story.

The Act provided that persons subscribing £50 or upwards would be eligible for election as vice-presidents of the hospital; a donation of 20 guineas earned life membership, as did the active collection of £40 or upwards. These positions carried voting entitlement in elections to Council at the AGM, as did an annual subscription of £2. A brisk business was done in award of these distinctions, certainly spurred by the shrewd policy of publishing the names of benefactors in the annual report.

The report accompanying the first AGM could list a growing surgical staff, now numbering eight. Three of these, Swanzy, Story and Benson, were described as surgeons, and Maxwell as junior surgeon, while four, Odevaine, Werner, Montgomery and Mooney were assistant surgeons. Nuances now, at that time such distinctions denoted a real hierarchy, as some still living can dimly remember. They all practised ophthalmology, and three at least were recorded as being aurists as well; in addition a Dr Hayes was listed as 'Physician for Diseases of the Throat'.

As the AGM would have been too large to accommodate in either of the hospitals, and the Lord Mayor being, ex officio, a member of Council, it was found convenient to stage the event in the Mansion House – which would be its venue for several years following. The expectant gathering learnt that of the minimum estimate of £30,000, only £16,700 had so far been collected. It was also announced that while a building site had not yet been obtained, Council was actively pursuing the search.

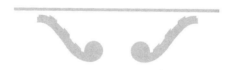

8

INSPIRATION FROM UTRECHT

Search for a site commenced with the appointment of a site committee consisting of two lay and two medical members of Council, answerable to the parent body. The latter positions were filled by Story and Swanzy as the ranking seniors in the new hospital. An architectural adviser being indispensable, Council chose the firm of Carroll and Batchelor which, temporary at first, was later granted the permanent title.

Effectively all dealings were with Frederick Batchelor. He had joined the office of James Rawson Carroll as assistant about 1892, and was later to become his partner. An Englishman, his first appearance as an authority on hospital design was in February 1897 when he presented a paper to the Architectural Association of Ireland on the subject of 'Hospitals'. Published in *The Irish Builder*, the communication, by calling attention to him as a coming man in a specialised field, was the likely cause of his engagement. The paper offered a workmanlike review of its subject, without frills or flourishes. In corresponding with the personality of Batchelor, a thorough worker with no worse foibles than cycling and the new craze of motoring, the paper would have served to endorse him as a steady man and to commend his candidacy.

The site committee remained in existence from November 1897 to June 1899. Although its ultimate recommendation was for the site where the

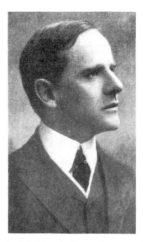

8.1 *Frederick Batchelor, when president of
the RIAI. As architect of the Eye and Ear
Hospital, he featured in a protracted dispute
over the builders' payment.*

hospital now stands – a plot already available and known to be so as early
as the committee's second meeting – the apparently barren intermission of
eighteen months was alive with activity of a sort which still can kindle
interest.

As to the areas automatically attracting first consideration, namely the
sites of the amalgamating hospitals, that of the National in Molesworth
Street could instantly be rejected as being too small. Lincoln Place was a
different matter. The land was owned by TCD and, despite constraints, it
seemed open to expansion if these could be overcome. St Mark's stood
neatly placed to the right of the back entrance of Trinity, its other flank
being delineated by a lane serving the rear premises of certain houses in
Westland Row. If this lane and some adjoining property, including a public
house on the corner, could be acquired and consolidated, it would present
a feasible plot for building or, more probably, expanding the existing
premises of St Mark's.

Batchelor quickly and effectively quashed aspirations to build upwards,
by pointing out that such a course would result in a building sixteen feet
higher than the nearby Dental Hospital and ten feet higher than Swanzy's
own residence in Merrion Square. After an initial misunderstanding,
delicate negotiation with Trinity College revealed that body to be not only
amenable but desirous to secure the hospital as a neighbour and tenant,
and an offer of tenancy was made on advantageous terms. But a major
difficulty intervened in the shape of an existing tenancy held by one

Captain Riall. This was not due to expire until 1904, before which the Trinity offer could not take effect. While some agreement seemed possible with Riall, the publican at the corner of Westland Row was likely to be obdurate. Records of the site committee show the heart-searching to have been long and painful before all thought of so happy a site was at last abandoned.

In the meantime, Batchelor had been inspecting other sites as they arose. In June 1899 he reported favourably on one in Adelaide Road, long available but only recently given serious consideration. Accepting the recommendation, Council forthwith instructed the site committee to buy it on the most reasonable terms attainable. The vendor, one J P Pile, offered to sell the entire plot for £3800, or else 250 feet frontage at the broad end (adjacent to Leeson Street) for £2800. Council opted for the whole plot, at the asking price if need be, but aiming to bargain for £3500 if attainable. Swanzy, and Lombard the honorary treasurer, were to act for Council. In the event they managed to get it for £3600, a deal endorsed with the hospital's seal on 10 August 1899.

An important part of this business has to be read between the lines. While events indeed occurred as minuted, it is evident that as early as May, the farseeing secretary had anticipated the eventual purchase of the Adelaide Road site, and accordingly took advance action to optimise the result. Swanzy was aware of several salient facts. First of all he knew that in Utrecht, Holland, the most modern eye hospital in Europe had been erected as recently as 1894. Secondly, a large international ophthalmic congress was due to be held in Utrecht on 14 August, at which most if not all of the Medical Board from Dublin would be present. So in May, realising that the Adelaide Road site was likely to be chosen, yet despite the absence of an agreement to purchase, Swanzy sought and obtained authority to organise for the architect to be in Utrecht in August at the same time as the Board members. Time was a factor where travelling arrangements were concerned; had he waited until June the necessary disposition of personnel might not have been possible. Small in itself, this incident goes far to show how in the overall pattern no detail, however minute, escaped the attention of the master planner.

Batchelor raised no difficulty and agreed to undertake the mission for a fee of two guineas a day, plus expenses. Should the Utrecht visit be in vain, he was allowed discretion to visit other continental centres in search of a model. In the event this proved unnecessary, and the ultimate account of his expenses came to a trifle over £40. It was to prove a valuable

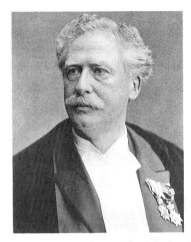

*8.2 Dr Herman Snellen, professor of ophthalmology, Utrecht.
His new Eye Hospital in that city formed Swanzy's
inspiration for the design of Dublin's 'Eye and Ear'.*

investment; the outcome of the Dublin party's visit to Utrecht was to be a milestone in Irish ophthalmological history.

To understand the ophthalmological significance of Utrecht it is necessary to regard the nineteenth-century development of ophthalmology into an exact science. In this evolution certain hero-figures stood at critical junctures, without whom the discipline would not have advanced as it did. Surgically there was von Graefe, whom Swanzy had assisted in Berlin; in optics and the whole huge science of refraction and accommodation there were Frans Cornelius Donders and Herman Snellen, successively professors of ophthalmology at Utrecht. Of the former Duke-Elder has written: 'Together with von Graefe and Bowman he was one of the great masters who guided ophthalmology in its earliest days into the maturity of an established branch of medicine.'

But in 1899 Donders had been dead for ten years, and the genial Snellen, his pupil and successor, was presiding in Utrecht. Almost of an age with Swanzy, he had together with Landolt revolutionised the clinical management of those needing glasses, incidentally gaining eponymous fame for the test-types that bear his name world-wide to this day. He belonged, in short, to the Ophthalmic Establishment, an invisible club of which Swanzy, by merit, was also an accepted member.

Snellen had occupied the Chair of Ophthalmology at Utrecht since Donders stepped down in 1877. It is clear that in him, as in Swanzy, academic excellence was admixed with administrative flair. Thus, under

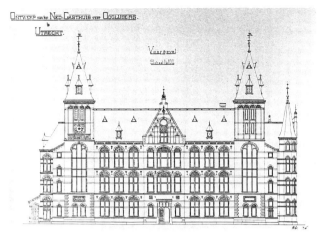

8.3 *Elevation of Snellen's Eye Hospital at Utrecht; signed
by Kruyf, the architect, it indicates a family likeness to
the style from which RVEEH was derived.*

his direction there had arisen the splendid new University Eye Hospital of
Utrecht, opened in 1894 and standing on a street where it would ultimately
be complemented with the unit honouring his predecessor, the F C
Donders Institute for Ophthalmic Research. A special bond of esteem
existed between Swanzy and Snellen. Reverence for the latter is shown in
Dublin to this day by the massive picture of him dominating the OPD
concourse in RVEEH since its inception. In counter-compliment, Swanzy's
ophthalmoscope is cherished in the Utrecht ophthalmic museum.

Given Swanzy's background of continental training, and his later
prominence in a chosen discipline, there is an automatic inference that he
kept open the lines of communication with his peers in other countries.
Here and there in his early history a glimpse of this academic intercourse
comes through, as happened that time when the British Medical
Association came to Dublin in 1887, allowing the coterie of distinguished
European ophthalmologists to express their 'high approval' on inspecting
the National. It was more than coincidence when, the following year,
Swanzy was chosen to deliver the prestigious Bowman Lecture, which a
century on still acts as herald of a coming star in the ophthalmic
firmament. Swanzy's subject was the value of eye symptoms in localising
brain disease, and his lecture presaged the ultimate tribute of presidency of
the Ophthalmic Society of the United Kingdom, which he held from 1897
to 1899. More honours would follow, but by now it was clear to all that

the Irishman shopping for a hospital in Utrecht was already a very important personage.

The building which had been opened in Utrecht on 9 May 1895 had been designed in 1891 by a local architect named Kruyf. He was a pupil of the renowned P J H Cuypers, whose work is familiar to many outside of Holland through the distinctive lines of the Rijksmuseum in Amsterdam. Both buildings favoured the neo-Renaissance style derived from earlier centuries; even as they were thus imitative, so too were they in turn destined to be imitated. Just as from Cuypers' Rijksmuseum followed some features of the same architect's Central Station in Amsterdam, so did his pupil draw upon the latter in designing his Utrecht Eye Hospital – the Nederlandsch Gasthuis voor Ooglijders. And this in turn was to become Batchelor's role model for the RVEEH in Dublin; indeed some traces of the same derivation are also visible in the Munich Eye Clinic, completed in 1905.

There exists no formal report of the architect's judgement. The absence of any written reference to the inspection, together with Council's subsequent unanimity that the right line was being followed, is eloquence enough. There is no cause to regard Batchelor as anything but his own man in reaching a decision, but the enthusiasm of the accompanying Board members on inspecting this shining-new hospital can only have helped to fortify his judgement. A brief minute of September, that Messrs Carroll and Batchelor had been appointed architects to the new hospital, is the only record of the momentous decision taken on 14 August 1899. Although the future form of RVEEH was conceived on that date it would take almost another five years in gestation.

9

BUILDING BLOCKS

For almost a year after the appointment of Carroll and Batchelor as hospital architects, there was superficially little movement with regard to building. But behind the scenes all was activity. The deal for the site was completed in January 1900 and a caretaker engaged. In the same month the architects submitted their plans, together with the estimated cost of completion, calculated at £41,500. To a Council permanently short of even the funds needed for day-to-day operation, the financial prospect must have been horrific. With a building fund standing at about £20,000 it pays tribute to Council's collective courage that after a month of shocked silence, instructions were given for working drawings to be prepared, and a firm of quantity surveyors was engaged.

Preliminary site excavation commenced in July, and eventually, a year and a half after the Utrecht visit, arrangements to engage builders were put in train. Selection was to be through limited competition, the winner to come from a list of firms drawn up by the architects. In respect of the main contract, of the seven firms invited to tender, only five responded, with quotations showing a variation of about £10,000 between the highest and the lowest. The tender chosen was the lowest, that of Messrs J & P Good of Great Brunswick Street, who quoted some £40,000 for the entire building and about half as much for a limited first stage. Additionally a

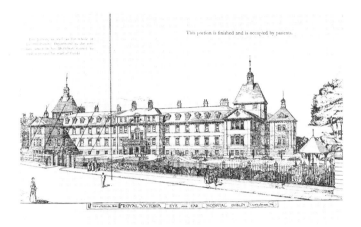

9.1 *Elevation of the proposed hospital drawn in 1901. This fold-out illustration, published at the expense of a Council member, showed the intended first phase (to the right of the vertical line).*

number of subsidiary contracts brought the first stage commitment to £25,000. Council ordered draft contracts for this stage to be drawn up with the successful firms, with J & P Good as the main contractors. It was a major decision, and one there would be reason to regret.

However, amidst the growing burden of expense and anxiety there were some gleams of encouragement. In the wake of the annual meeting of 1901 came a letter from Mr Wellington Darley of Bray, a contributor of notable generosity, and already a vice-president for that reason. He promised £500, equivalent to perhaps £10,000 today, towards the stipulated target of £30,000, whenever the latter sum would be 'made up', thus in a neat package managing to exalt the Victorian virtues of both liberality and self-help. Some time later, through Dr Peacocke, Church of Ireland Archbishop of Dublin, an anonymous contributor, later revealed to be Colonel Trench Gascoigne living in Yorkshire, offered £1000 on condition that a further £4000 be raised during the following six months. When this inducement still failed to raise the nominated sum, the time limit was extended for six months more, the donor finally settling that the money could be handed over, provided that only the interest on it would be used until the target had been reached. Here Mr Wellington Darley intervened, authorising payment of his £500 if doing so would satisfy Colonel Gascoigne that his conditions had been met. The latter was agreeable, and so ended this engaging sort of set dance, seemingly designed to make munificence self-multiplying.

At about the same time a member of Council, Mr Justice Andrews, offered to pay printing costs for a sketch elevation of the projected new building, for inclusion as a fold-out in each copy of the report, running to a circulation of 8000. This was so popular that he later funded a further printing of 10,000 copies for use in publicity. The picture was a handsome line-drawing showing the finished design in black and white, with the yet unattainable portion hatched in red. It still has an attractive eye-catching quality that reveals the generous man of law as a good judge in more than his professional capacity.

As to building operations, from the very start relations with the firm of Goods were beset with problems. The Good brothers were master builders, still remembered in the trade, but in the present context the historical researcher never encounters them face to face. The view obtained is always glimpsed through some medium, be it letter or lawyer or arbitrator. A constant impression is that just as some people are accident-prone, so with the Goods there was ever a new crux, an uncharted hazard. Even before the contract was signed, they failed to have the draft ready in time for Council's perusal at a stated meeting. As a result an extra meeting was required, a lapse which won Council's displeasure.

Within a month another cause of discord had arisen. The new difficulty was over a security bond that Council wished to have embodied in the contract, to cover any defects or deficiencies arising in the workmanship. However, by the time this issue was raised the draft contract had become effective, and Goods declined to enter into any guarantee other than what was specified in it. Here they were within their rights, so that on legal advice Council cast about, seeking private insurance. This was destined not to be realised, but such an outcome was not anticipated prior to Goods' tender for the work being accepted, on 14 June 1901.

When it became clear that there would be no insurance the fat was in the fire. For over two years until November 1903, when the architects took over the finished building, there must have lain at the heart of Council business a lurking unease at this lack of guarantee. Such latent insecurity could only increase with a disaffected, and ultimately hostile, builder.

Ill-will showed itself in September 1901, some three months into the contract. Goods wrote asking Council to nominate an arbitrator to decide questions in dispute between builder and architect. This request was declined by Council, which held that power of ruling on the disputed issues lay within the architect's professional competence. In conveying this opinion to Goods, Council sternly enjoined them to proceed actively with the building works at Adelaide Road, which Council understood were

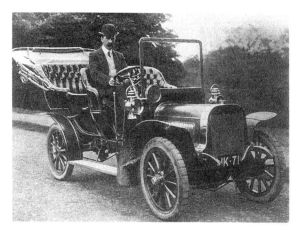

9.2 *John Good, head of the firm that built the hospital. A contemporary account described him as 'stormy petrel of the building trade in Dublin'.*

being 'delayed, if not at a standstill'. Goods complied reluctantly, stressing that they did so under protest and reserving the right to future claims for compensation, a stance Council immediately repudiated in writing.

This unhappy relationship fretted on for the next two years until Stage One of the contract had been completed. The main bone of contention lay in Goods' constant importunings of Council for payment, a demand as constantly met by Council's response that payment hinged on the architect's certificate of work properly done, and that such certificates were not always forthcoming. At this remove in time analysis of all the factors is no longer possible, but there certainly was a head-on confrontation between builder and architect in October 1902. The latter reported to Council that, whereas slates on the operating block were being secured in an unacceptable way, and wooden sills of some of the dormer windows were split and should be replaced, the builder had refused to rectify these defects when instructed. The building committee sought legal opinion as to whether the architect was entitled to withhold his certificate, and his action in doing so was endorsed, a decision resolving that particular issue, which is not further mentioned.

Whether the basic trouble was a personality clash between the Goods and Batchelor rather than bad workmanship, is a matter of conjecture. The building has worn too well for defect of workmanship to have been fundamental. It is obvious that Council's attitude to the bickering was consistently correct; moreover the Goods undoubtedly lacked sensibility of the relationship proper to dealings between architect and builder. Against the argument that they were difficult individuals who often appeared provocative is the fact that their agitation was sometimes justified, as when an outstanding £4000 was left unpaid for want of certification. It was well they could not foresee a final certificate of more than treble this sum!

All of this detail would hardly be worthy of record, had there not come in May 1903, news of an impending royal visit, featuring the new King, Edward VII, and Queen Alexandra. At all times corporate loyalty to the Crown was a marked feature of Council's outlook and circumstances where such loyalty was in chime with the hospital's advantage offered an ideal opportunity to blend instinct with expediency. There had been a previous flutter of enthusiasm in 1900, when on the rumour of a visit by the then Prince of Wales it was resolved to ask him to open the hospital. That visit had proved to be a private one, but now the advent of a new reign offered opportunity for an illustrious opening. A letter was drafted asking that His Majesty might be pleased to visit the hospital and perform a short ceremony, and evidence indicated that a favourable answer was expected.

In anticipation of this desired event, Council wrote requesting the Goods to make such arrangements in finishing parts of the new building as were necessary in view of the probable visit of their Majesties. Goods replied that they would do so, provided that Council would assist in resolving the difficulties between them and the architects.

Predictably, this put paid to a royal opening. Since Council could not comply with the condition, the Goods countered with a downright refusal of the request. Council's bright hopes were dashed and the optimistic imaginings plummeted. A letter from the Viceroy to the President of Council summarises the end of this spiteful episode. He wrote: 'I had submitted your letter to His Majesty and I think that he was disposed to visit the Eye and Ear Hospital during his stay in Dublin but in view of what you now tell me I will substitute the name of some other institution for His Majesty's consideration.' On this sour note did the Goods achieve what was at best a hollow victory.

Settlement of the storm in a teacup was next attempted through arbitration. This involved a new character, one James Beckett, who volunteered to act as conciliator and was recommended by Batchelor as an honest broker. At the time James Beckett was senior in a well-known family building business, partnered by his nephew Bill, later to be father of the playwright Samuel.

James Beckett had in fact been one of those originally asked to tender

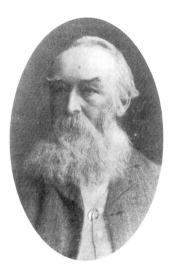

9.3 *James Beckett, sometime president of the Master Builders'
Association, who acted as mediator in the dispute over payment.
Head of the prominent firm which built the National Library, he
was a grand-uncle of the playwright Samuel Beckett.*

for the RVEEH contract, when his figure had been second highest. It is
possible that his re-entry at this stage was instigated by Batchelor who had
first nominated the panel of builders and would now have been anxious to
resolve the impasse at almost any cost. However, by this time Council,
cautious of all builders, would only deal with Beckett at one remove, his
letters all passing via Batchelor. Before his mediation would be accepted
he was asked to obtain from Goods a full list of all monetary claims and of
matters unresolved with the architects.

Meantime the hospital, conscious of a large outstanding debt, had
sought Counsel's opinion on its situation relative to the Goods, who by
now at white heat, were demanding interest on unpaid money and even
imputing to Council a capital gain of dividends through non-sale of
investments. This unworthy allegation was speedily repudiated. Eventually
the skirmish was succeeded by a sullen truce, and in the end, after the
architects had certified the payment of £13,000 owing to the Goods, the
building was handed over by the contractors in November 1903. The only
beneficiary of the argument appears to have been Beckett, who having
entered the case as a genuine mediator seems in time to have become the
heir-apparent, inheriting any business arising after the Goods had
departed.

A coda to the whole unhappy affair appeared many years later when, in April 1911, on Batchelor's advice, a payment of £600 was made to Goods in final settlement of all claims, this being Council's limit of compromise in a deal to be rid of the firm for ever. Yet before they vanish from notice, it is no more than justice to accord the Goods, as builders, the credit which has accrued to them in the light of history. After nearly ninety years of existence and despite the assaults of many modifications, their fundamental work remains sound as oak and as likely to survive for many generations.

The builders vacated the site in November 1903. Yet, though the edifice was completed, all the work of equipment and furnishing lay ahead, together with the thousand details of what effectively amounted to creation of a new institution. It was not until 18 January 1904 that transfer of the first patients, from the National, took place, to be followed one month later by those from St Mark's. The Royal Victoria Eye and Ear Hospital had been a legal entity for nearly seven years, albeit under two roofs. From 18 February 1904 it was a physical reality, under the single roof that shelters it today.

10

ABOVE POLITICS

While it is a truism that by its nature a hospital should be an institution above politics, it is no less true that the nature of humanity demands a political dimension in most of its institutions. When the amalgamating hospitals found the necessity to produce an identity that society would recognise, their histories presented no great difficulty. In their separate foundings each had been guided by a similar ethos, based largely on the established Church and the Crown. Though by 1897 the Church was no longer established, the structures still obtained, and in general RVEEH was, and was perceived to be, a pillar of the accepted order. An ascendancy still prevailed, and by and large the hospital was an extension of that ascendancy.

Indeed the dimension of loyalty to the Crown as a factor common to the uniting hospitals had probably helped in settlement of their unfortunate disagreement as to naming. Since each of them had lost a cherished title, the 'Royal' prefix would certainly have been a consolation prize to loyal subjects. Other loyal gestures were not lacking, such as Council's order for verbatim entry in the minutes of the letter permitting display of the royal arms; and the prized gift of a large framed photograph of the Queen. Such things, so trivial now, were then obviously seen as part of the fabric of the foundation.

In keeping with them is a minuted item authorising Beckett to erect in the grounds a big free-standing flagpole, to be hinged at the bottom. A contemporary picture shows this object erected before the East Front, where it would certainly have served to display the Union flag on suitable occasions. It is surprising therefore to discover a letter written by the registrar in May 1904 and addressed to Sir A E Vicars, Ulster King-at-Arms, the authority on heraldry in Ireland (a name known to later history as official custodian of the Irish Crown Jewels when they were stolen). Parker's letter asks him to view and authenticate a flag 'purporting to be the national flag of Ireland' which Council had ordered as hospital regalia. It showed a golden harp bearing the bust of Hibernia, against a pale blue ground.

The answer to this request is not available, but the episode underlines the eternal anomaly of the Crown in Ireland, since it indicates some sort of identity crisis even in those distant days. Both of the flags referred to are still extant, keeping amiable company with the Tricolour and the Papal Arms as evidence of ready adaptability and generations of careful housekeeping. The flagpole has disappeared long since and no one now remembers it; however, as appendix to this story, documentary evidence shows that in 1907 it was accidentally broken by a firm of painting contractors. Accepting liability, they proposed to repair it by splicing but were denied this outlet by a Council intent on reinstatement.

There had always been, especially in Wilde's foundation, a recognition that the charity existed for all the people. To this effect he had from early days striven to ensure that his hospital would not be denominational, and from the 1850s on, until the death of Wilde, the names of Dean Meyler and Dean O'Connell, successive parish priests of St Andrew's, Westland Row, were to be found featuring on the committee of St Mark's. It forms no part of the hospital's history to investigate the social background to the change in practice after Wilde's death, when this ecumenical gesture was abruptly withdrawn; it is possible that disestablishment of the Church of Ireland, coming about that time, served to close the ranks of its adherents.

A wry repercussion is echoed in the National's minutes of 1897, just prior to amalgamation. A Catholic lady from Donnybrook had asked permission to visit and read to the patients in the National. The Governors were amenable to the request 'if arrangements could be made to separate those of different religious denominations, so that the reader, of whatever denomination, should only be able to address his or her co-religionists'. This strait outlook led to the farcical situation that while the first readings were reported to have pleased the patients, 'the Protestants did not wish to be excluded from the room during the readings, indeed strongly objected to being so'.

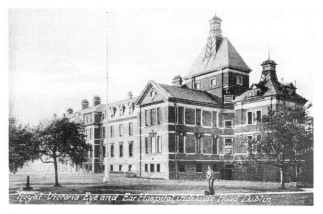

10.1 *East Wing and Entrance Block, shortly after completion.*
Note the flagpole in the foreground.

As a result, the Governors were on the point of sanctioning a mixed audience, when an over-prudent voice suggested that to avoid possible offence the matter be referred to the Protestant chaplain. He compounded the issue by providing a special reader for his own flock. The sorry affair precipitated one of the earliest RVEEH Council decisions, ruling that no lay person might visit the hospital for the purpose of reading to patients.

The sagacity of this resolution is surely traceable once again to the temperance of Swanzy, without whom no policy decision of any moment was made during his lifetime. Unlike St Mark's, the National with which he was identified, had never featured clergy of any denomination on its committee and in turn this came to be an unwritten character of the new hospital too. Similarly, in December 1904 a Council resolution ordained that (merely for identification purposes if required) the religion of each house-patient was to be entered in the admission book and nowhere else. Perusal of the roll of Council members shows that a measured attempt was made to impart a 'mix' of persuasions in its composition, with the establishment retaining a discreet majority. From this distant view it was no doubt seen as a fair arrangement that those of education and means should still keep sway over institutions founded by themselves or their ancestors.

Perhaps it was even the best solution possible for that time in history. The medical faculties of Trinity College and the College of Surgeons had for decades and even centuries produced graduates imbued with the confidence born of long tradition. The National University had not yet been born, and the infant medical school of its immediate predecessor, Newman's Royal University, was still learning to find its feet. Hence, book learning apart, the graduates of the older foundations were endowed with the unteachable asset of 'know how', thus making them uniquely qualified to preserve continuity of tradition. Furthermore, in the spacious early years of the century, with the Boer War a receding diversion, the menace of the Kaiser only a shadow, and the idea of insurrection not even that, the decades of Victorian peace and prosperity must have seemed likely to go on for ever. The mood was not ripe for change. It looms as one of the more intriguing exercises of this study to trace how, despite these facts of history, within the present century the public image of RVEEH has altered and its climate been transformed, while yet its informing spirit of succour has persisted unchanging.

It is appropriate here to notice how over several decades RVEEH and the Adelaide Hospital enjoyed a sort of syncretism, Swanzy being the common factor. Except for a short break (1876-80) when teaching demands deflected him to the Dr Steevens' Hospital Medical School, Swanzy's association with the Adelaide was continuous from 1870 until his death in 1913. Cherishing the same values of Church and Crown which he held dear, the Adelaide was in a sense his spiritual home, and also gave him safe anchorage where nursing matters were concerned. Certainly a number of his nurses at RVEEH were derived from its excellent School of Nursing; it was from the Adelaide that in 1908 the redoubtable Miss Reeves came to RVEEH as matron, she who would later leave so firm an imprint on the founding articles of the General Nursing Council of Ireland (An Bord Altranais today).

There was thus mounted a *mise en scène* of potentially great complexity. On the one hand the Adelaide, of avowedly sectarian charter, on the other RVEEH, humanitarian in outlook and dealing with universal specialties wherein confessional argument was unlikely (though not, as we have seen, impossible!). In between stood Swanzy, steadfast indeed in his persuasion, but nonetheless unshakeable in the vision that for Dublin and Ireland the best course to chart would be a non-denominational foundation for the special senses. Two thousand years ago when Horace wrote of erecting a monument more lasting than bronze, this was only to prefigure the triumph of Swanzy's achievement. For today, approaching the tenth decade since its building, his hospital displays not alone the bronze tribute decried by the poet, but exhibits in its own fabric the monument that endures.

On the ground, as its *genius loci,* Swanzy was untiring. His constant influence can be discerned in the records, which in addition to Council minutes include a pair of letter books covering the first decade of the century; taken together these documents offer a close-up view of the

hospital's activities as it evolved. Unfortunately, the available archive deter-
mines that, although voluminous, the records are necessarily one-sided,
since for any given situation a detailed statement of the hospital case is apt
to be balanced by a sketchy outline of the contrary point of view. Only too
often this is left to the imagination, the absence of responding documents
coming as an anti-climax when the scent seems at its strongest.

Nevertheless, the sharp picture emerging is notable for its consistency.
Central to the archive is the figure of Edward Parker, appointed registrar at
the amalgamation, and proving himself a diligent officer of the hospital.
Although he lacked a role in the process of decision-making, this history
owes him a debt for more than seven hundred letters, written in a clear
hand and invariably lucid in their message.

As well as revealing certain once-off situations attending the launch of a
new institution, the correspondence shows other themes to be perennial.
Whether in subscription-raising or debt collection, the topic of finance is a
constant; more than anything else this predominance gives the flavour of
what courage and enterprise were required of the founders and
proprietors of a voluntary hospital. Above all it is seen that careful
watchfulness as to every penny was the cement enabling the concept of
the voluntary hospital to cohere.

In the letter books, the pitch of correspondence was liable to reach
high gear if the stakes were commensurate, as when for instance the substantial Weir Estate came to be distributed at the discretion of its executors.
The benefice was confined to Dublin hospitals, among which, though a
new arrival, RVEEH featured as an eager claimant and certainly not the
least deserving. Since a dignified prospectus was essential, presentation of
the hospital case demanded the use of a typewriter, then a rare accessory,
still the last word in office equipment. Consequently a machine was hired
at a cost of 7/6d a week and employed to state at length the hospital case.
The happy result was an allocation of £3000 from the fund. Apart from the
Cyclopia Bazaar and the Gascoigne Incentive this major benefaction rates
as the largest single source of funding for construction.

The tone of certain letters is redolent of the period, though this may the
more reflect personal mannerisms of the registrar than the attitude of
Council. All the same it falls strangely on modern ears to find a Lord Mayor
of Dublin being addressed as My Lord, just as the acknowledgement 'very
obediently' of Dublin Corporation's substantial annual grant of £275 seems
somewhat craven to the reader of today. There was a regular traffic in
correspondence with the Poor Law Unions about contested accounts. Not
all of the Unions were 'good pays' and the registrar's pained letters carry

complaints as to cheques out of date or entered for the wrong amount. Seemingly the banks had not yet devised the euphemistic 'refer to drawer' and the ultimate indignity of the bouncing cheque was indicated by a terse N.F., meaning no funds were available to meet it. The usual penalty in such circumstances was refusal to admit further cases from the offending district until an advance deposit was credited to the hospital; the sum of £5 was usually considered sufficient guarantee of renewed solvency.

The contrast with our modern system, computerised and studded with projections and estimates, is extreme. Whereas today's overrun of expenditure is generally if not invariably met from central funds, in those earlier times the onus of making ends meet lay on the individual or committee. The result was a more intimate operation, conducted as an exercise between individuals, each offering to the other a face, a personality and feelings capable of mutual interaction. Although Swanzy is represented in his obituaries as being somewhat cold and distant on casual acquaintance, this austerity hid not only a kind heart but also an iron will. This last was the driving force which powered the hospital, aided by a willing Council and a multitude of helpers on the ground. Collectors were active in all parts of the country, their efforts recognised in the many pages of itemised acknowledgements in the annual reports.

Another recurring theme was a protracted arbitration with city opticians, both individually and as represented by the Irish Opticians Association. From this long perspective come echoes of trade rivalry between firms aspiring to identify with the hospital, and the efforts of their association to implicate Council in the matter. The latter, determined not to become a party to commercial competition, decided to rotate the concession at yearly intervals between the various claimants while reserving to medical staff the right of independent recommendation. But the rivalry still simmered, eventually being brought before the finance committee of Dublin Corporation as warden of the hospital's annual grant. After a satisfactory inspection of the hospital the latter offered alternative recommendations; a shorter term of rotation, which Council found acceptable; or serial rotation of the appointment through all candidates, which Council declined, as such a mandate would infringe its independence. The end-impression gained is that of a cautious Council holding aloof from a commercial issue charged with strong feelings. However, in personal terms, Council's attitude to opticians was distant to a fault. Responding to a questioning patient, the registrar wrote: 'It was a mistake for Messrs X to write to you, as the attending optician sinks his personality for the time being, and is here merely "the optician".'

Strong feelings of another kind were apt to surface on the subject of vivisection. In December 1907 a regular supporter, Sir Gilbert King, declined his usual subscription having been informed that vivisection was practised at the hospital. The affronted Council approved Swanzy's reply asserting the utterly unfounded and practically impossible nature of the charge. Miss Beaufort, a collector for many years, demanded and got removal of her name from life membership of the hospital for no reason other than the discovery that Dr Swanzy was a member of the RDS 'which seems to have a great admiration for vivisection'.

Woven in with letters offering a serial narrative, there are hundreds more giving a fleeting glimpse of other aspects of life in the early century. Post-Victorian business practice was little changed from that of earlier times and small frugalities were still rated a virtue. Examples of fund-raising, internal economies or just plain begging abound in these pages, offering quirky alternatives to administrators in this age wherein the voluntary idea has been so sadly superseded.

For example, when long before its time the idea of a joint laundry was circulated to some dozen hospitals, only two of them, RVEEH and the Coombe, were receptive. For lack of support the project languished, but RVEEH had shown willing, and is seen to emerge with credit. A printing firm remiss in revising proofs of the annual report was advised that if the published report were to contain any serious error in printing or finish, the account for it could not be passed for payment. And when a cricket ball from the College Park came through the window at St Mark's, it eventuated in a stern letter to the police.

Since typewriter hire lacked a long-term future, purchase of the hospital's very own machine eventually became incumbent. Enquiry as to price was followed by a letter naïvely hinting that the London makers might perhaps see fit to present a model free of charge. It was suggested their reward could be found in good publicity among the numerous hospital subscribers whose names were listed in the report enclosed. Unsurprisingly, the ploy was not successful, and most regrettably the reply has not survived. The final choice of an Empire machine was a decision of such moment as to justify notifying the suppliers that there would be no deal unless covered by a six-year guarantee.

This miscellany of written papers shows the new institution as not merely an amalgam, but also as a body animate of itself. Like any living organism, whilst owning to its parentage, it bore distinctive and unique characteristics of its own. The growth and development of these comprise the remainder of this story.

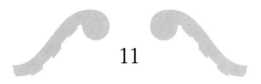

11

'COMMODITY, FIRMNESS AND DELIGHT'*

It has never been asserted that Frederick Batchelor was among the greats in architecture, nor in justice would he be likely to have so represented himself. Chief assistant to Rawson Carroll from the early 1890s, he later became a partner in the firm and was effectively the active member in all dealings with RVEEH. Since the disagreements with J & P Good touch so closely on this history and because inevitably they lead back to Batchelor, it is more than idle curiosity to enquire both as to his competence and to whether he too had a difficult personality, leading to mutual antagonism with the builders. Fortunately, a short biographical sketch exists, written by Frederick George Hicks, another Englishman, eventually to become his partner on Carroll's retirement. While such an account is likely to be pre-judged in Batchelor's favour, the impression gained is that of a sound man, agreeable in person and professionally so well esteemed as to attain presidency of the Royal Institute of Architects of Ireland during 1908-09.

Hicks writes of him as a rapid and clever draughtsman and admits to being lost in admiration at his ambidexterity, telling how he always wrote in pencil with his left hand and in ink with his right. At work his energy was prodigious; he mapped out a programme for each day and adhered to it rigorously, no matter how late the hour of its fulfilment. On a lighter note he mentions Batchelor's achievements in cycling, which included a circuit of Lake Geneva in a single day, as well as possession of a hundred-mile certificate. Later he took to motoring in a steam car of eccentric behaviour, known as the Yellow Peril. In it he was reputed once to have taken eighteen hours to travel from his home in Greystones to his office in Dublin. These enthusiasms mark him precisely as a man of his time, cycling being still identified ·as the cult activity of the 'naughty nineties', while the famous Gordon Bennett Motor Race of 1903 is an Irish landmark of motor-sport in the early century.

During the seventeen years they spent as partners, Hicks tells that only once did he and Batchelor have a serious disagreement, which he generously accepted as having been entirely his fault and following which they were better friends than ever. This sketch is doubly useful, both in exonerating Batchelor from being unreasonable and in describing the precision of his work-practice. The latter is possibly the needed clue as to the root cause of disagreement between such a methodical, literal-minded Englishman on the one hand, and the Good brothers on the other, master craftsmen surely, but probably resentful of taking orders from one they regarded as a 'blow-in' from across the water. However it may have been, a confrontational ending was all the more regrettable since it had been Batchelor who at the outset had nominated the short list from which the builders were chosen.

The paper on 'Hospitals and Hospital Construction' read by Batchelor to the Architectural Association in February 1897 could not have been more timely for his interests: it has to be seen as the direct cause of his firm's retention by the site committee. In this paper he classified hospital design as comprising four categories – pavilion, block, corridor or a composite type designated the 'heap of buildings'. Whatever his personal preference, the final drawings would inevitably have been influenced by the visit to Utrecht.

At this point it appears suitable briefly to regard *fin de siècle* architecture in Holland, especially as touching the eye hospital in Utrecht, designed by Kruyf, former pupil of the renowned Cuypers. In the later nineteenth century, under the influence of Viollet le Duc in France and of Pugin in England, the architects of Western Europe had tended to look back to their medieval roots. As a result, various derivatory styles had emerged, known severally as neo-Gothic, neo-Renaissance and, drawing randomly from both, a composite style called neo-Eclectic. All of them found favour in Holland, especially the neo-Renaissance mode, recalling Dutch architecture of the seventeenth century. A typical feature of it was the brick façade interspersed with courses of natural stone, a sandwich of white between layers of red, which the Dutch called speklagen or layers of fat. Typical also was the capping of window openings with alternate round and triangular hoods, a device inherited from Palladio. In addition, the use of keystones was common, and roof edges were often made of natural stone. While richly decorated surfaces are noted as another feature, in deference to the functional nature of hospitals this was omitted as inappropriate in the present instance.

The style adopted for Utrecht showed neo-Renaissance elements to be predominant. One classification rates it as neo-Eclectic, a hybrid name offensive alike to ear and eye. Meant to suggest a culling of the best from all periods, if only for euphony this clumsy term is to be avoided, and in reference to RVEEH the term neo-Renaissance will be preferred. While both hospital ventures were ambitious, the project in Holland had surely been less daunting than the Irish one, having University backing, whereas almost every penny raised for the Irish hospital had to be got from private pockets. Some resultant economies in RVEEH will become apparent.

The design finally agreed for Dublin embodied three stories over a basement and presented an 'H' plan carrying pavilions on both halves of each perpendicular; the horizontal bar housed a main corridor and various other accommodations. The first phase envisaged completion only of the East Wing (nearest to Leeson Street), together with the entrance block and eastern corridor, so that the 'H' figure would still lack some of the crossbar and any part of the left perpendicular until funds would allow.

From the outset it had been decided there was to be no extravagance in respect of decoration, either within or without. This principle was observed in general; happily it did not entail the loss of good taste, which was destined to befall so much hospital building later in the twentieth century. Conforming to the style described above, the principal element of the design was a red brick façade, divided into registers by horizontal limestone courses in line with the window openings, and crowned with a mansard roof of green slate, pierced by attractive attic windows. A contrasting keystone gave added liveliness to the first floor windows, and the attic ones were graced with alternate round and triangular hoods in the Palladian manner, albeit made of wood. The pavilion gables, facing forward, were endowed with a brick pediment featuring a circular window with keystone ornaments.

Centrally, the façade was permitted to break forward to accommodate the main entrance. In celebration of this the doorway was marked by a *porte cochère* supported by four rusticated stone pillars, and surmounted by a balustraded surround incorporating the royal arms.

With so positive an assertion on the ground floor, an answer from the façade above was demanded. This took the form of a Venetian window flanked on each side by overlapping giant pilasters of the Ionic order. Topped by two large limestone scrolls simulating an open pediment, the entire feature ran vertically through the three top storeys. The name and date of the hospital were blazoned in gold along the frieze.

Of all the exterior features displayed by the new building, few will disagree that the lateral towers form what is probably its single most striking aspect. With contours showing a strong family resemblance both to the Rijksmuseum in Amsterdam and the hospital in Utrecht they bring to Dublin architecture a flavour unique in the city's manifold styles. The green-slated hipped roofs rise in a high pitch to chisel-edge ridges, straddled by wooden turrets and ending in a flèche. These vertical markers indicate the junctions of main corridor with the pavilion wings lying at either end. But there is more, for the annexes prolonging the main building are similarly capped on a diminished scale, adding in a single stroke both echo and endorsement of the overall design.

Time has dealt not unkindly with these features, especially the *porte cochère,* which in retrospect can be seen to have arrived as the ultimate statement of an age already expiring. Even as Batchelor was designing this portico for the coach-borne, he himself with his steam car was writing an epitaph for the coaching age. In practice, while the facility for coaches would have been seldom used for the ostensible purpose of its design, it must undoubtedly have sheltered, as they waited, the many humble suppliants for admission who had never known the grandeur of coach travel. However, its real destiny still lay hidden in the womb of time. It must be seldom that something which marks the end of an epoch manages to acquire a new function in the succeeding age. Such was the destiny of this quaint windswept appendage, when early in the seventies it was adapted to serve as a much-needed entrance lodge and telephonist's station. Since the original plan had signally failed to provide a reception area, this neat amendment has happily cured the deficiency.

The fact that Batchelor's design derived, via Utrecht, from a medieval revival movement, places RVEEH squarely in concert with Europe's late nineteenth-century school of architectural thought. In the further role of a purpose-built eye hospital it embodies dignity of another order. Although stipulated to be kept free of florid ornamentation it yet has a personality proclaiming good ancestry. It ever remains inspirational that Ireland's largest eye centre is a scion deriving dually from the rootstock of European

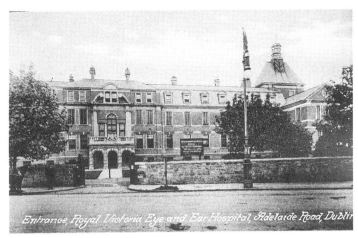

11.1 *The original Entrance soon after building. Access from the*
street lay opposite the front porch.

continental tradition, and that it was built for the purpose it continues to
serve.

Swanzy shared with Wilde a feeling for history, and just as the latter
had welcomed ancient traditions in taking over the charity of St Catherine's
Hospital, Swanzy too was conscious of following an admired example. The
large portrait of Snellen, described as dominating the out-patient concourse
in RVEEH, is a token of his homage. There is evidence that another visual
feature was available which, for whatever reason, he forbore to use.
Lacking documentary evidence the case remains unproven, but at the least
it deserves mention in offering a possible further insight into Swanzy's way
of thinking.

Unlike the unadorned entrance at RVEEH the main doorway to the
Utrecht Hospital had a series of symbolic mural decorations. As well as
plaques indicating dates of first founding and re-establishment, there were
a number of allegorical images referable to ophthalmology, figures of
dragons standing for danger – hence disease, obelisks for constancy, and
above all that of a rising sun, the epitome of light. The cipher for the latter
exactly duplicated the astigmatic fan invented by Snellen as a diagnostic
aid in eye testing and still in use today. Iconographically, the last named
therefore had double significance, to acclaim the allegorical source of light
and to emphasise the hospital's role as a centre for diagnosis.

Both of these motifs had an obvious attraction for Swanzy, who had
long since shown himself open to appeal by allusion. This had been seen
in his regular use of the picture showing blind Tobit as cover feature on

the National's annual report, along with Goethe's apt quotation; likewise with the classical topic he and Fitzgerald had chosen for the RVEEH seal.

The question therefore arises as to why he should have failed to seize on the rising sun motif which held attraction for himself and honour for his friend Snellen. Two answers suggest themselves. Firstly, that to imitate Utrecht in this feature might have smacked of plagiarism, or else, and more likely, that Swanzy felt bound by his promise to avoid extravagance in a building erected by the hard-won funds of his subscribers. As a man of honour he would have scrupled frivolous expenditure, as some might have thought it, even though it would favour his personal preference. If this interpretation is correct, it arouses added admiration for the self-discipline of Swanzy. Knowing his form, it is possible to surmise a struggle of warring emotions between the student of tradition and the man of honour, and to admire the latter's victory.

Externally, the original approach for pedestrians is now effaced completely. It lay along the shortest possible path from Adelaide Road to the main entrance, and is discernible in an early photo. The paved carriageway came much later. The early years embody a saga of attempts to beautify the grounds with trees and shrubs, and overcome the double disadvantages of soil polluted by builders' rubble, and of the Adelaide Road climate, subject to east winds blowing along the canal. Many hours of thought by Swanzy and letters from Parker were devoted to this problem, but alas, their genius for administration was not matched by gardencraft, and the *naïveté* of some queries to nurserymen is hilarious for lack of elementary horticultural knowledge. Indeed in gardening matters all commonsense seemed to desert these two normally shrewd guardians of their fief. This was seen when a cheque for plants to be delivered was cashed by the gardener, who then kept the money! But their legacy of trees and greensward survives, no mean bequest in this age of the voracious motorcar.

---

*The chapter title is a quotation from Sir Henry Wotton's *Elements of Architecture* (1624). The full version reads: 'In architecture as in all other operative arts, the *end* must direct the Operation. The *end* is to build well. Well building hath three Conditions. Commodity, Firmness and Delight.'

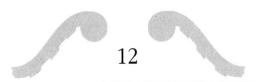

12

BEHIND THE FAÇADE

Since the hospital was constructed in at least three stages, with over twenty years between opening and completion, a difficulty naturally arises in treating of the 1904 interior. It is unlikely that anyone now living can remember the scene greeting the visitor in its early years. Hence the account that follows has to be read in the knowledge that, written with hindsight, it describes the architect's visionary interior, not fully completed for two decades.

Before visiting Utrecht, Batchelor's original view as to layout had been that while a block pattern would be cheaper to build, a design featuring a central corridor was operationally preferable. The design at Utrecht endorsed the latter, and accordingly when his plan was revealed it showed a long straight passage running from east to west without interruption on all four floors of the building. However, by 1904 only the Entrance and East Wing with connecting corridor were completed.

The arrangement was simple and in the main effective, suffering only from the defect of its virtues, which was that the basement corridor, assigned to services and not patients, was externally accessible only from the rear, and internally from the ends of other corridors. This led to an upstairs/downstairs situation occasionally comparable to a maze. Rationalised, the underlying idea was excellent in that it contrived to sever

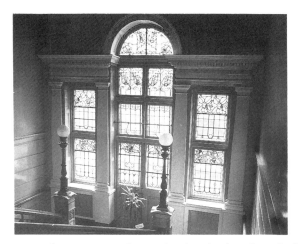

12.1 *View of Venetian window on landing leading from the hall.*

non-medical activities such as cooking and laundry from the patient areas. In practice however, by isolating the entrance door from everything else on its own floor the quirky effect it produced sometimes amounted to bewilderment.

To the first-time visitor confusion was pardonable, when just past the front door he found himself confronted with a substantial granite staircase going upwards, flanked by blind alcoves going nowhere at all. In fact, this curious arrangement presented two sides of the same coin: on the one hand a disembodied entrance, on the other, an ingenious cleavage between medical and domestic activities. Only with assimilation of the *porte cochère,* already described, was the entry integrated into the functional unity of today.

Once up the stairs the gracious Entrance Hall became apparent. Backed by three windows containing small leaded lights of opaque glass with art nouveau decoration, it formed a central node on the long east-west corridor behind the façade. Upwards from it twin flights of stairs doubled back towards a handsome Venetian window occupying the south wall and flooding the whole space with light. From the landing thus formed the two stairways resumed the climb in a single flight supported by two painted Doric columns based on square pedestals in the hall below.

The hall flooring consisted of a marble chequer of black and white squares in the classical style. At the foot of each staircase stood the respective doorways of Registrar's Office and Council Room, while as it entered and emerged from the hall the corridor was announced by arched apertures housing swing doors with attractive small pane glazing. As traffic

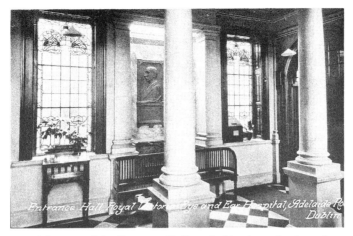

12.2 *View of the Entrance Hall, probably about the time of World War I. The bronze memorial to Sir Henry Swanzy is visible.*

has multiplied it is regrettable that these handsome doors now tend to pass almost unnoticed, being permanently pinned open by day.

From a contemporary photograph it appears that the bust of Sir William Wilde, donated by Story, was mounted in the place of honour, resting on a plinth seated on the central window sill. In front of this stood an elegant mahogany seat of unusual design, long since transferred to the Council Room for safety. It is here suitable to mention that after Swanzy's death the central window embrasure became literally a niche of honour, site of a marble recess with bronze plaque recording his dates and exploits. The bust of Wilde is mounted nearby, and this record chooses to revere them as equals in the role of Founder.

As to what the new building contained, at a remove now of some ninety years, the most reliable insight comes from contemporary sources. At the AGM of 1904, held just after the building was occupied, Council's mood was not merely jubilant but euphoric. In the brave new world just created, every novel feature called for emphasis; the sophisticated external venetian blinds, wound by elegant brass fittings from within the wards, were singled out for special praise. Made of wooden slats and intended to relieve eye patients from the glare of sunlight, these lasted many decades until they were finally replaced by conventional roller blinds. Simpler in function, the substitute lacks the quaint appeal of the 'period piece' original.

On the other hand, the provision of gates at the end of each corridor to prevent blind or partially sighted patients from falling downstairs, represents a fixture as valuable today as when erected. Hanging superbly despite their width, the solidity of these gates is a source of pleasure as constant as their recorded cost is a surprise. The sum of £8.3s.0d. appears to represent an inclusive figure for two gates in the wing then completed, a bargain indeed for such workmanship. Other cause for boasting in 1904 lay in individual bell-pushes for each bed, as well as internal telephones and both passenger and food lifts. These accepted features of our time represented advanced technology for their day, although performance of the lift will call for further mention. As for the large Day Rooms, vitally necessary for the many ambulant yet long-stay patients of 1904, these have been subsumed to other use in the changed conditions of today.

Two Operating Rooms were provided, 'well lighted towards the north'. The Nurses' Home on the top floor was 'very perfect' with separate bedrooms. Below, stairs, kitchens and sculleries were spacious and well-lighted, and besides a range there was the means of steam cooking as well as a soup-boiler and milk-steriliser. Also proudly noticed was a tea stillion: unknown today, it turns out to be a cradle for supporting a vat or tea urn. All of this equipment was procured without incurring debt, in great part thanks to a bazaar specifically organised to raise funds for furnishing.

In an effort to emulate the success of the original Cyclopia Bazaar this function was given a name which, meant to be distinctive, succeeded only in being outlandish. In a derisory attempt to cap the pun of Cyclopia, this function for the 'Eye and Ear' was named the 'Ianer' Fete and Bazaar, and held in the hospital during the first five days of December, 1903. However much the naming may have been a damp squib, when the receipts came to be counted they produced a satisfactory bang worth £1500.

Treated as a major social occasion, the bazaar's thirteen stalls and eight side-shows were given several pages of coverage in the next report. The vital trigger of competition had been touched by a promise to publish not only the names of stallholders but also their takings. A decided sense of period is preserved in the naming of stalls, such as the Bon-Bon, the Bric-a-Brac, the Poikilos – a medical borrowing meaning 'of many sizes' – and the Omnium Gatherum. Side-shows featured a ballroom with dancing to Herr Feddersen's Band, a *café chantant* and an area of unspecified activity called the Fish Pond. As to receipts, the Poikilos stall under Mrs Swanzy was a clear winner with £216, matron coming second with £174 and Mrs Batchelor third with a respectable £160. Miss de Groot with her palmistry took just £10, while the Halls of Laughter, featuring contorting mirrors, returned a mere £6.8s.3d.

Behind almost every aspect of equipping and furnishing stood the watchful presence of Swanzy, directing here in person, there by committee, often through the registrar. Insurance of the building had to be arranged, being finally divided between three firms, each bearing £7000 worth of cover at an annual cost of five pounds per company. A large order for 'aseptic hospital furniture' was offered to Down Brothers, the London instrument makers, but subject to stipulations. Would they send a man to unpack? Would they guarantee to replace any article damaged in transit? And confidentially, would it be all the same to them if the order were to be given them through a Dublin firm, and if so, which firm would they advise?

General furnishing and its trimmings gave scope for a tireless search for perfection. The minutes note that Council delegated the choice of furniture for the Council Room to the discretion of Messrs Swanzy and Benson. The letter book seems almost to suggest that for a while Swanzy laid aside his usual unobtrusive role of grey eminence, to assume that of commander in the field. Thus there is at times almost an imperious note, as of orders given in the heat of battle. Witness the registrar writing in March 1904: 'I am directed by Mr Swanzy to say that he mentioned best American cloth for the chair covering, which is cheaper than hair cloth and preferable to it. Please send revised quotation accordingly.' Or again, Swanzy in a note to Batchelor: 'The estimate for the dumb waiter seems much too high. Kindly obtain one or two others. I think canary wood enamelled would be nicer.'

Even recent observers, knowing the hospital only for a short time, will recall the ward tables in daily use until lately and still extant. Solidly tile-covered they stood, familiar and all but indestructible; it still comes as a surprise to discover that their design was no thing of chance but the formal choice of a founding committee. The decision to have green and primrose tiles of specified size and pattern reads like a birth certificate, spurring fresh recognition of these day-to-day objects as authentic originals, part of the stuff of history. A similar authenticity attaches to the gaunt and extremely uncomfortable examination chairs still lurking in the Out-Patient Department. Not yet quite discarded, to generations of patients and doctors these furnishings were inseparable from the practice of the department. For teaching purposes they doubled as easels, housing in their straight backs a moveable board capable of being slid vertically upward for casual use as a blackboard. The unique thrift of these dual-purpose articles qualifies them as perfect museum pieces.

Furnishings apart, there was much still to do before the building would be completed. A brusque note from the registrar to Beckett in May 1904

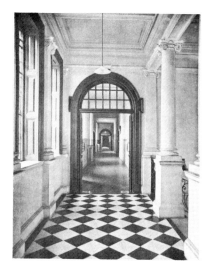

12.3 *A second floor corridor, soon after opening.*

conveys some sense of the partly organised chaos that reigned at this stage. This letter delivers Swanzy's instruction that estimated work must be kept quite distinct from jobbing matters. 'There are several things left half-finished in the dispensary which cause inconvenience and Mr Swanzy wishes the men engaged on these and other occasional jobs to complete the work in hands, without being taken off – as he frequently finds – to assist at contract work.' Still mining the letter book, another nugget to surface is an extract spelling out Swanzy's exact wishes to a firm of joiners, ordaining that should their estimate for certain articles be accepted, they will be required to submit a proof item roughly put together before being finished off, and before the remainder of the order is completed. Happy times, when the customer was always right!

But even as the rose is subject to the worm, so before long inner flaws in the building began to search out its stamina. It was true that like the poor, certain problems were perennial – the Goods for instance, who for years yet would be grumbling about payment; or the unpainted plasterwork which required a two-year drying-out period before allowing of decoration; or the missing units of West Wing and Out-Patient Department, both still unbuilt for lack of funding. Such burdens were facts of life, and thus in the short term acceptable. Trouble with the tiles and with the lift were unexpected and called for remedy.

About a year after opening, ominous ailments appeared in the tiling, especially on the landings where faulty workmanship resulted in tiles becoming loose or hollow sounding, while a manufacturing defect was shown by chipping and signs of surface wear, at a time when the product was barely a year in position. Fortunately the episode involved no fresh grapple with the Goods, tiling not having been part of their contract. However, before it was disposed of, delays caused a series of skirmishes with the English manufacturers, their Dublin agent and the tiler, adding to the pains of management and restricting efficient functioning of the hospital. One letter read: 'The grit from the cement bed treads all over the place, making an unsightly mess, and has practically ruined the black and white marble over the entrance hall. The black marble is covered all over with dirty white scratches and will never look the same again.'

The rebuke was merited; defacement of the pristine marble flooring, that rare concession to elegance, must have indeed been galling. Happily the incident lacked the malice found in dealings with the Goods, and the matter closed with no cost beyond the annoyance. In the tile context, there is a feature in the corridor tiling which breathes artless sophistication, and has always impressed this observer as advanced practice for 1904. This is the smart and functionally useful 'coving' entailing a line of concave tiles marking the junction of side walls and floor. The simplest of devices, it entirely eliminates the trapping of dust and debris endemic to such areas if they are right-angled.

In the early twentieth century the passenger lift was still a prized novelty even in a public institution. In engineering circles, the rival merits of hydraulic and electrical power systems had not yet been determined. In 1904 both were valid options and Batchelor's selection of water power rather than electricity was bad luck rather than bad judgement. Unfortunately it was to provide a major snag in the new building.

Intimations of supply difficulties had arisen during planning. In December 1902 Council noted the demand likely to be made on the Corporation water main in Adelaide Road. The specification was for a four-inch pipe to supply fire hydrants in the grounds and a three-inch one for the hydraulic lift. The Corporation initially responded that a two-inch pipe was the maximum allowable to any public building, but two months later relented, allowing a three-inch supply for the lift. So far, so good. In practice however this supply was found to provide only enough power to raise half the expected load, with all the attendant inconvenience. An appeal to the Waterworks Committee was a vain one from the outset, since the recently piped Vartry water supply, though prized by Dubliners for its drinkability, lay in quiet storage in the reservoir at Roundwood, without prospect of substantial pressure variation. In addition, defect of the lift mechanism required repairs to the hydraulic cylinder owing to continuous leakage, so that what should have been a boon, instead proved a constant handicap.

By 1908 the hydraulic system was so inadequate as to stimulate enquiry about the electrical alternative. In December 1908 the registrar was asked to write to the BMA, in whose London premises a staff member visiting from Dublin had been much impressed with the arrangements for elevation. Always a great questioner, Mr Parker was here in his element. What firm had supplied the lift? Was it electrical from the start or had it been converted? And if you don't mind me asking, what did it cost?

The answers are not available but clearly were satisfactory. The hydraulic system had been found wanting and the speed of its abandonment has to reflect the direness of the situation. By February 1909 Council had approved conversion to electrical operation at a cost of £411. Apart from minor hitches, there was no further trouble in this department, and costly though the conversion was, it was probably regarded as cheap at the price.

13

EXCELSIOR!

Despite settling-down problems inevitable in a new building, by 1907 it could be claimed that under tight management, the domestic finances of RVEEH were on a sound footing. The cost of subsistence was less than 8d a day for each patient, while yearly bed cost was a little over £41 per bed unit, less than one third of the rate in other hospitals. Bed occupancy showed the increased hospital capacity to have been fully justified. Correspondence responding to a circular from Sir Charles Cameron, the City MOH, revealed that unlike the generality of hospitals there was no rotation of ward closures. Instead RVEEH was kept going at full capacity the whole year round. Despite this, from time to time there was such demand on beds as to provoke longing looks towards the day when the residue of building would be completed.

Meanwhile there presented a more pressing need which was inescapable. Daily to be seen at the most sensitive interface between doctors and patients was the lack of any formal area for out-patient examination. As a makeshift, the basement space intended for a laundry was being used for everyday clinical examinations, resulting in congestion quite out of keeping with the spacious accommodation upstairs. Of the two main causes for continuing space deficiency, perennial lack of funds was probably the lesser. A greater nightmare loomed in the still unsettled account of the Good brothers, which stalked the pages of Council business for the best part of a decade and inhibited further building.

The balance of legal opinions on this issue, and there were many, was in the country phrase, 'to let the hare sit', the inference being that it would run when it was ready, or otherwise was likely to grow old and die. Council remained at all times willing and indeed eager for a fair settlement, but Goods continued to nurse their grudge rather as a child hugs the rag doll it hates to part with. Minuted evidence suggests that Batchelor was the Goods' main target through refusal to issue the final certificate. In an effort to disengage itself Council required him to relate independently to the builders in the light of his professional status, also declaring its inability to permit the hospital's solicitors to advise him. But to no avail; the Goods remained as a sort of moral picket for far longer than reason might justify.

In this way Council's wish to build an Out-Patients was dogged both by the unfinished settlement and by an uneasy fear that Goods might bring a law case, should a fresh contract be made with some other party. Despite advice that the contract with Goods was binding only for five years from the original signing, progress was desultory between 1907 and 1909, although an intention to proceed was evident through preparation of plans and an advertisement for tenders. In 1908 the Board of Superintendence for Dublin Hospitals endorsed the need of RVEEH in a plea advancing the particular role of out-patients as a social grouping. 'They are as a rule, persons who though disabled by chronic ailments, try to hang on to their work. To attend to them quickly and efficiently and let them go their way is a great charity.' This appeal gave a fillip to the raising of funds and in 1909, with half the calculated cost of £10,000 collected, a contract was signed for erection of OPD premises. There still remained Council members who feared a reaction from the Goods if building proceeded, but their fears were allayed by a series of cautious resolutions hedging the stance of Council and clarifying it for posterity. At the final vote there was only one dissentient.

The plans had been drawn by the new partnership of Batchelor and Hicks and the successful tender was submitted by the firm of J and W Stewart. James Beckett, who might have been expected as a contender, did not appear even in the short list, and he may have died by that time. The last mention of him in any context was in 1908. Although the hospital continued to do business with his nephew Bill Beckett, the father of Samuel, the old sense of personal commitment was no longer there. James Beckett's departure from the scene makes it timely to pay tribute to the definitive role of peacemaker which he played at a time critical for the hospital.

J and W Stewart ran a no-nonsense firm committed to getting on with the job. They commenced work in 1909 and with no discernible check, had finished by the end of the following year, the out-patient building being occupied in January 1911. In advance of this a subscription ball in aid of the furnishing fund was held in the building itself, realising the useful sum of £139. The estimated building cost of £10,000 happily proved excessive by some ten per cent. However, with a deficit of still almost £3000 the hospital's Micawber-like situation persisted.

What had now been acquired was a free-standing annexe, with an extensive ground floor and a rather smaller upper storey in the part distal from the main building. Grandiosely claimed by Council to be 'the finest Out-Patient building of its kind in the Kingdom' it provided ample space for the almost 40,000 annual extern attendances hitherto dealt with in the basement. Open-plan arrangement being in favour at that time, the huge rectangle of floor was divided essentially into five spaces. The whole of one end was occupied by a reception area where charts were issued and patients' destinations decided; under a large glass roof its counterpart at the other end combined an open-plan refraction room having five separate eye-testing stations sharing common floor space with one another and with the 'waiting' benches on the sidelines of activity. Between these two ends, the still large space remaining was divided into three, providing on either side the makings of bright and spacious clinical units. In the centre was a core common to both but lacking independent daylight. This housed a darkroom with multiple cubicles and adjacent stairs to the upper storey.

This storey was home to ENT out-patients and a small laboratory; it comprised several large examination rooms as well as two smaller units supplied with running water and equipped for minor surgery. It has undergone much mutation in the course of years but has never relinquished its original prime purpose as the ENT enclave. Additionally it now houses the medical social worker's office, while the laboratory area has overflowed to accommodate the National Ophthalmic Pathology Laboratory.

In train with these advances, there flits through the archive a wraith of day to day hospital activity in the early century. The random glimpses on offer show a way of life insulated from today by two world wars and a scientific revolution. Though the items presenting to the researcher are truly miscellaneous, a strange unity invests them, all reflecting facets of the same complex organism.

In 1904, the year of opening, Council made early show of its charitable bent with the order: 'That the word "Free" be printed on the white prescription papers used in the dispensary, and that the several members of the medical staff be written to, requesting issue of those papers to decidedly poor patients only; and use of the blue papers in all cases where patients can pay the few pence chargeable for the medicine.' While this epitomised the ideal which informs the social conscience of all voluntary hospitals, sadly, within two years it became necessary not only to beg the prescribers to draw rein, but also to ask the Medical Board to determine whether the dual system of dockets should continue at all. Whether or not it did matters little at the end of the twentieth century, but at RVEEH there still survives from previous times a rubber stamp marked 'Free' wherewith needy patients could be identified at the pharmacy.

The slowly changing social order is marked by the appearance for the first time of women resident doctors. Dr Kathleen Lynn – whose story comes later, in another context – seems to have been the first. In 1907 a Dr Thomasina Georgiana Prosser displayed her feminine disposition for home-making in a letter complaining of the lack of a sittingroom in which to receive a friend. Council responded by offering use of the Council Room in the afternoons, except on Tuesdays, when it was occupied by the ladies' sewing guild, and the Registrar's Office in the evenings. This deficiency of accommodation would finally be made good with completion of the West Wing.

Dr Prosser was clearly a woman of spirit, befitting her pioneer role. Being constrained to attend court by subpoena under the Employer's Liability Act, she protested the duress. The recorder upheld her, ruling that he would not order any professional person to give expert evidence without a professional fee being guaranteed them. Council saw fit to enter this decision in the minutes.

During that same period there was reported the mournful news of a house-surgeon's death while in office, the cause unstated. Dr Sibthorpe was assuredly a scion of the decorating firm of the same name which shortly afterwards secured the contract for painting the hospital. Despite the bereavement touching both parties, the business arrangement remained, but evidence of friendly goodwill was noted in the contractor's proposal to donate to hospital funds £10 from the agreed contract total.

A minute attention to detail indicates how tightly run was the administration, clearly illustrating the old definition of genius as being an infinite capacity for taking pains. Once the great enterprise of the new hospital had been launched, it was unquestionably this painstaking

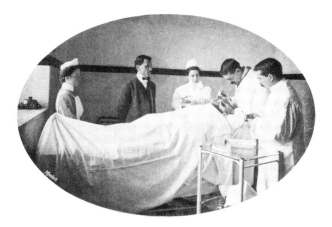

13.1 *Theatre scene in the new hospital, c.1908.*

capacity which kept it going; it is likewise certain that the genius was Swanzy's. While the meticulous Parker proved an able executor he was at all times carrying out policies conceived at a higher level. The letter books furnish multiple examples of his style in stewardship, and a few may be cited.

The need for stringency dominated all other considerations, at times to a fault, as when the hospital needed a sewing-machine and someone suggested that if approached the makers might donate one. Erection in the grounds of a noticeboard appealing for funds was a matter in which Swanzy took an active personal interest. A letter from the registrar to Beckett cites in detail Sir Henry's precise wishes both as to the legend required for the board and the size of letters to be used. The concluding line, 'I hope this is quite clear', brings to mind a distinct impression that Parker, the writer, foresaw himself as Sir Henry's first target if anything were to go wrong and that he was anxious to avoid this role if possible.

On one occasion he is seen to write to a coal merchant complaining of the 'excessive quantity of dross' in a supply of steam coal, the consignment having consisted largely of coarse coal dust incapable of making a blaze; if the suppliers could not improve on a rival offer of small Welsh steam coal at 14/- a ton, they were likely to lose the business. It seems that indeed they did lose it, for the following year's complaint was to another merchant. Its topic varied also, featuring the surprisingly modern theme of the 'perfect fog' of smoke produced by a supposedly smokeless coal. 'This is an important matter for us; it not only incenses the neighbours but has an injurious effect on the young trees and shrubs in the grounds.'

Soon after the official opening, similar concern for the hospital's appearance was evident in a letter to the secretary of the Dublin Tram Company, complaining that a company delivery van had used the carriage drive instead of the goods entrance specially provided. Parker had personally witnessed how the driver had carelessly cut into the grass edging with a wheel as he left. He forthwith reported the incident to the company, notifying them that trivial though it might be, he would have to debit them with the cost of repair. The excuse that the driver was unaware of the goods entrance was not accepted, as in any case he had been seen to effect the manoeuvre deliberately sooner than await the removal of an obstructing vehicle. Quite apart from an understandable chagrin at defacement of brand new premises, there is latent in this correspondence the young century's respect for the propriety of law and order, a concern too often absent in this, its last decade.

Parker's role in fund-raising was central, the more so as his terms of appointment secured him a percentage on certain monies raised by his own efforts. Probably as a result, the intensity of effort spent on this activity was prodigious. For years before and after the new building was opened annual reports were voluminous with acknowledgements of individual subscribers. The funding campaign was based on counties, and sums as small as 3d were given individual mention. Collecting boxes played an important part and were issued wholesale. C E Fitzgerald had one in his waiting room but was tardy in returning it; when opened in 1908 its contents were found to include a cheque dated 1905, for the sum of one pound. It was drawn by the Rev Thomas Moore, a regular subscriber; in asking for its re-validation, the diligent Parker ventured a reminder that the current year's donation was still outstanding.

So, by steps small and large, the new hospital began to loom as a presence on the Dublin scene, and be seen by Dubliners as an institution ever ready and dependable. As for Swanzy, however much the patriarchy of such a foundation might seem to be self-sufficient, this was not so and he sustained a host of diverse activities. As the most renowned oculist certainly in Ireland, and possibly in the two islands, his practice was, at the least, demanding. Running through many editions, his textbook on eye diseases required constant revision, eventually needing the editorial help which he found in Louis Werner. As he thus toiled on untiringly, his deeds were not unnoticed by the profession. In other disciplines his peers, conscious of the giant in their midst, were searching among their treasures to see how best to salute him.

The Dublin establishment was first to act, when the Council of RCSI paid him its highest surgical honour, electing him president of the college for the years 1906 to 1908. He was the first ophthalmic surgeon ever to attain this distinction, in which a decade later he would be joined by the faithful Story. But in any age, hospital founders come thin upon the ground, and Swanzy's total achievement was sufficient to call for still more recognition. So it was that during his presidency he was also granted a knighthood. This brace of distinctions became multiple when in the same year the University of Sheffield saw fit to confer on him the honorary degree of D Sc.

Thus with his life's work acknowledged, his cup was full for all the world to see. But as long as the West Wing remained a draughtsman's dream on paper, he still lacked the last measure that could bring it to brimming.

14

NEMESIS

Fate is seldom even-handed, and close on the heels of so many honours, Swanzy suffered the death of his wife in 1909. Other than the conventional expressions of regret no word of his personal sorrow appears in the records. It is rash to attribute feelings in what is an historical record, but hard to avoid a conclusion that this reminder of his own mortality could not fail to act as a spur towards completion of his life's work.

The Out-Patient building was such an immediate success that after one year's operation a twenty per cent increase in attendances could be reported. However, there was to be no resting upon laurels. Notice of the improved attendance, made at the AGM of 1912, was almost simultaneous with the announcement that an additional eighteen beds would be added by building a portion of the West Wing, at an estimated cost of £5,000, the existing complement of eighty-two beds being too few. Despite Lord Iveagh's generous gift of £50,000 to Dublin hospitals about this time, the RVEEH share of £2000 was already largely bespoken, so that there was virtually no money in hand for the new venture.

Where then were funds to come from? Previous example had always shown Council as prudent almost to a fault, but this time it was content to express trust in the benevolence of human nature, indicating past results as evidence. A keener reading would suggest that, fearing indefinite deferral

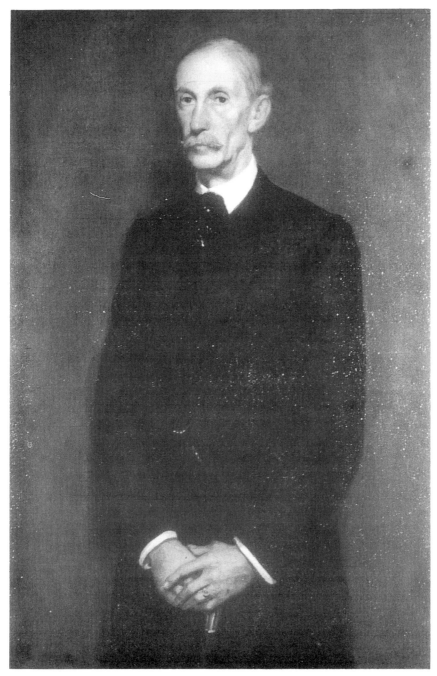

14.1 *Portrait of Sir Henry Swanzy, painted by his daughter Mary Swanzy.*
Reproduced by kind permission of its owners, the Board of the Adelaide Hospital.

if Swanzy's guiding hand were no longer available, Council decided to press on with the work while there was still momentum, or in the racier language of today, to 'go for broke'. It is conceivable that Swanzy himself recognised a perverse logic in this, and conscious of 'time's winged chariot hurrying near' relaxed his usual caution.

The decision once taken, a quick choice was made from a selection of plans advanced by the newly formed firm of Batchelor and Hicks which, already apprised, had several alternatives in waiting. The venture in all conscience was relatively modest, envisioning westward extension from the centre block, adding corridors plus adnexa, but stopping short of the West Wing that would complete the building. There was no delay in work starting; it commenced in September 1912, although the famous strike of 1913 was to delay completion. This organised labour unrest was just one of many signals that the world in which Swanzy had grown and so notably flourished was about to vanish for ever.

In his personal life, the passing of various younger colleagues and co-workers so soon after his wife's death could only have been a sombre reminder that herein he had no lasting city. The death in July 1912 of Robert Montgomery, one of the assistant surgeons, was quickly followed by that of Arthur Benson in November. Though he had been ill with heart trouble for more than a year, Benson was all of a decade younger than Swanzy, and the loss of this longtime friend must have represented real grief to the older man. Hardly was he cold in his grave when in January 1913 there followed the death of Edward Parker, Swanzy's alter ego in the pages of so many letters on hospital business. The last tribute to this staunch administrator told how Council 'held Mr Parker in the highest esteem and regard for his integrity of character and devotion to the hospital which owes him much for his services since its foundation'.

Other changes marking this new decade included Lloyd George's Insurance Act of 1911, with its complex knock-on effect on hospital administration, and two medical staff appointments bearing omens for the future. These 1912 harbingers of the changing face of practice were the specific assignment of Dr T O Graham as clinical assistant in care of nose, throat and ear cases, and the almost imperceptible metamorphosis of Dr Euphan Maxwell from the grade of house surgeon to that of curator, a grey assignment that could lead to better things. The case of Dr Graham foreshadowed the birth of separate departments for ophthalmic and ENT cases under the same roof. That of Dr Maxwell coming in the heyday of the suffragette movement could hardly have been more topical, since chrysalis days ended, she would soon emerge as the first woman ophthalmic surgeon in Ireland.

Although 1913 had a mournful start in the death of Edward Parker, and indeed showed an unwelcome portent of war in the stockpiling of fuel, these gloomy tidings did nothing to deter promotion of a special appeal introduced by Swanzy early in the year. The mood was that despite calamity the noble work must be seen to continue. Amongst Council's business at this time several items may be instanced. A new registrar, George Howell, was chosen to succeed Parker. Through negotiation the bank was induced to grant the half of one per cent discount on the loan rate for the new building, a measurable concession at that time. Dr Euphan Maxwell was advanced from the post of curator, subject to a cautious rider that appointment as clinical assistant was not to be regarded as giving any claim to further advancement on the staff ladder. But while in these divers ways the hospital was signalling its undisturbed equilibrium, destiny had ordained otherwise. On 12 April 1913, like a bolt from the blue, came the death of Sir Henry Swanzy.

It stole upon him in the form of a scarcely regarded attack of influenza, which progressed to heart failure, the whole taking a mere five days from onset to conclusion. It came so abruptly that many of his friends knew of his illness only on reading of his passing. At the time of his death, he was in his seventieth year, having been born in 1844.

In every sense this was the end of an era. On the personal plane it closed the career of an individual of high talent and absolute dedication. Professionally it marked the cleavage between the pioneer ophthalmologists of the nineteenth century and the new men of the twentieth. Nationally and internationally it found Ireland poised at the respective hinges of world war without, and armed insurrection within, events destined to swing shut the doors on British Ireland and the leisured Europe of the nineteenth century.

For all these reasons Swanzy stands a Janus, looking before and after. Contemporaries rightly accorded his death the importance befitting the passing of a really great man, although two world wars and an amazing technological revolution have conspired to blind later generations to this greatness. It is remarkable how up to now no biographer has arisen for so eminent a subject. Accordingly, at this crossroads it enhances our vision to view how he was seen and eulogised by those privileged to know him.

The shocked Council which met on 15 April unanimously passed the resolution forming the only business of the meeting: 'The President and Council of the Hospital desire to place on record their deep sense of the irreparable loss which has been sustained by them personally, and by the hospital, in the decease of their Honorary Secrctary, the late Sir Henry Rosborough Swanzy. The hospital owes its origin almost entirely to his initiative and public spirit, and the presently existing excellence of its structure and organization is largely to be ascribed to the unremitting personal attention which he devoted to every detail. It was through his loyal and single-hearted efforts that the many difficulties surrounding the amalgamation of the two older hospitals were surmounted through the Act of Parliament obtained in 1897. Since that date he never spared himself in seeking to arouse in others his own enthusiasm on its behalf, and in promoting its development and improvement in everything that modern science could suggest. This hospital was the great aim of his life, and it stands today as a lasting and worthy monument to his memory.'

The shockwave of loss reached far beyond the circle of Swanzy's immediate associates and far beyond the Irish shore. Much though he figured in the public eye, Swanzy was essentially a private person, and any sketch of him would be incomplete without some selection from the personal views of his contemporaries.

Having listed his achievements, the obituarist in the *British Medical Journal* went on: 'Sir Henry Swanzy was a man respected by all, but his real character was known only to his intimate friends; behind a veil of modesty and shyness, which was apt to give the impression of brusqueness to those who did not know him well, was a rich sense of humour, a warm heart, and a great charity, always ready in private life to find excuses for those who failed. The writer of this notice can vouch for the truth of the following story, which was typical of the man. A medical student who went to consult him about his eyes asked him his fee. Sir Henry said, "Nothing; dog don't eat dog". "Oh," said the student, "I'm not qualified yet; I am only a student". Sir Henry's reply was, "Neither does dog eat puppy". In public debate he was unsparing and scathing to any whom he suspected of humbug and dishonesty of purpose, but with the honest striver, however inefficient, his patience was inexhaustible.'

The London ophthalmologist, Sir Anderson Critchett, his friend of forty years, wrote that Swanzy's death broke one of the few remaining links with Donders, Bowman and von Graefe. Swanzy had greatly valued his association as assistant to the last-named, a remarkable genius whose memory he held in lasting and profound veneration. Critchett described Swanzy's textbook as 'one of the most excellent handbooks extant on diseases of the eye' and referred to his Bowman Lecture of 1888 as 'one of the best in that brilliant series, combining originality of thought and expression with diligent and successful research'. In personal evaluation he wrote: 'It was impossible to know Swanzy without loving him, for with the highest qualities of intellect and character, he combined a warmth of heart and a store of genial wit which attracted and held fast all who came within the range of his friendship.'

Among all the eulogies, that of C E Fitzgerald, his friend since student days, is unique in its author's close association with Swanzy for most of their joint lifetimes. Published in the *Dublin Journal of Medical Science*, and forming a source document for many of the details of Sir Henry's career, as a personal tribute it stands alone. Of Swanzy's social qualities he claimed to speak with an authority founded upon their close intimacy over so many years. He said that joined to a natural reserve of manner there was in Swanzy a certain nervous self-consciousness against which he seemed always to be fighting, but which in later years he had got under marvellous control. These factors led to an erroneous impression shared by many, that he was cold, indifferent and unsympathetic. No idea could be more mistaken; behind this exterior lay a warm heart and an affectionate nature, and above all a tender conscience. Though veiled by an apparent stoicism, these traits were all the more real through lying deep and being revealed to few. Added to them was a keen sense of humour and quaint originality as a raconteur.

While his main monument is the RVEEH, Swanzy left another in his *Handbook of Diseases of the Eye* which, first appearing in 1884, was immensely popular among students, no less in Britain than in Ireland. It reached thirteen editions, the last appearing in 1925. In the later editions Swanzy collaborated with his younger colleague Louis Werner (Senior) who, in addition to work on the text, enhanced the book with beautifully executed paintings of the ocular fundus. The framed originals now hang in the Research Department of RVEEH. Thanks to the spontaneous generosity of Louis Werner (Junior) during his lifetime and the willing co-operation of Mrs Werner even in our shared time of loss, it has been found possible to include a colour reproduction of the delicate artwork in this book.

While there was universal recognition that the hospital itself was his monument, Swanzy's stature was such that his admirers felt the need to demonstrate their esteem in public expression. The mobilisation of parties interested in erecting some more intimate memorial turned out to be altogether remarkable, and took shape in a meeting announced over some of the most illustrious signatures in the land; starting with the Lord Mayor of Dublin these included the Lord Chancellor of Ireland, the respective presidents of the Incorporated Law Society, the Chamber of Commerce and both Royal Colleges of Physicians and Surgeons in Ireland, along with four peers of the realm, Meath, Monck, Ardilaun and Pembroke. The gathering held at the Royal College of Surgeons in Dublin, on 3 July 1913, produced a unanimous resolution that a permanent memorial should be erected in Dublin to the late Sir Henry R Swanzy, which should, if possible, take the form of completing the Royal Victoria Eye and Ear Hospital, to the foundation and construction of which so much of his life had been devoted. Subscriptions were invited towards the sum of £12,000, calculated as requisite. The mounting of a personal memorial in the hospital was envisaged.

By way of enlargement on this announcement there was published a List of Committee, 3 July 1913. If the previous list had been star-studded, this one was a veritable constellation, for it named all those who had signified the intention of promoting Swanzy's memory by contributing to the memorial fund. The list was distinguished not only by names prominent in Ireland and Great Britain, but also by an immense array of ophthalmologists from abroad, numbering at least one tenth of almost three hundred names. Originating from Rome to Stockholm, from Paris to Vienna, they included admirers from places as widely scattered as Budapest, Cracow, Heidelberg, Upsala, Pavia, New York, Berlin, Hamburg, Zurich, Prague and other names unspoken.

For ophthalmologists this list has a unique lustre, constituting a galaxy of names seminal to the specialty. Included are those of Morax and Axenfeld, Birsch-Hirschfeld, Doyne, De Lapersonne, De Schweinitz, Elschnig, Fuchs, Gullstrand, Haab, Hess, Kuhnt, Leber, Landolt, Mellinger, Nettleship, Parsons, Priestly-Smith, Schmidt-Rimpler, Schiotz, Schirmer, von Szily, von Hippel and Vossius. To any Irish reader of ophthalmic history few of these will fail to strike a chord of recognition as pioneers in the discipline, or a glow of satisfaction that in H R Swanzy they acknowledged the existence of a peer.

The personal memorial was erected in the Front Hall of the hospital where it can be seen today. Unveiled in October 1916, it stands as perpetual reminder for generations to come that RVEEH did not happen by accident. Indeed not by accident, nor by State action, nor by any circumstance save the inflexible will of one man, wherewith he inspired a multitude of others to such efforts as would accomplish his vision and safeguard their own.

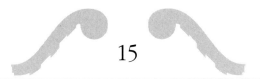

15

THE WAR CALLED GREAT

In every way but in actual dating, the death of Sir Henry Swanzy marked the watershed between the centuries. The seventeenth annual meeting of RVEEH, held in March 1914, epitomised the cleavage. On the one hand, less than a year after his death, Swanzy had already become part of the stuff of legend; on the other there yawned the imminence of World War I, after which nothing would ever again be the same. The 1914 meeting, probably the most liberally annotated of the entire series, brought reverberations of this changing world.

Suitably recognising the dual loss, to Council of its inspiring genius, and to the hospital of its secretary, the report announced Story's succession to that position. Due to the 1913 strike, progress on the building extension had been delayed, but at last completed, was due for occupation just as the report was issued. The addition created a building debt of over £5000, secured by a bank overdraft which would long cause anxiety. A total of over 1500 in-patients was the highest on record, as also were out-patient attendances in the region of 50,000.

While deficiency in income was deplored, a significant feature of the accounts was that although the usual subscriptions from corporate sources such as the Dublin Dockyard and Hammond Lane Foundry continued, the demise had occurred of another regular subscriber. Quite simply, as a result of Lloyd George's Insurance Act of 1911, the Great Western Railway

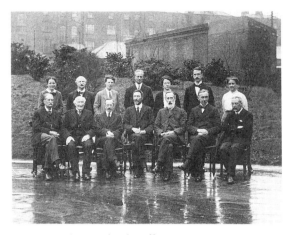

15.1 *Medical staff group in 1915.*

Society had passed out of existence. To a seer, had one existed, its passing carried a clue comparable to the biblical cloud no bigger than a man's hand. For thus, even before the Great War, a far-off bell was tolling for the voluntary hospital system, as structures arose which would determine the State's future grasp on the purse strings of medicine.

In the wake of Swanzy's passing, staff changes were inevitable. Their speed of accomplishment was swift as it was startling. With Story's enhanced status as sole senior surgeon and also secretary of Council it was foreseeable that the knock-on promotions of L J Werner and H C Mooney would follow. This left two vacancies at the bottom, one of them being predictably filled by R H Matthews, already for some time a clinical assistant. It was the other vacancy which had explosive potential, as Dr Euphan Maxwell, daughter of a member of the senior staff, was a prominent and most suitable candidate. The issue likely to be in contention was not that of nepotism, which indeed did not arise, but the fact that no woman had ever previously been elected to staff membership.

The same meeting of the Medical Board which recommended R H Matthews stated that owing to Dr Maxwell being a woman, it hesitated to recommend her for a similar appointment, while fully recognising her personal and professional suitability. The Medical Board accordingly sought Council's advice in the matter. In the first instance Council adroitly side-stepped the challenge, by directing that the vacancy be advertised. However, by the time of its next meeting opinion had crystallised and there was unanimous agreement in favour of the lady's acceptability, the appointment being ratified without further ado. In this way, an issue which in other theatres might have smouldered for months or years, became by

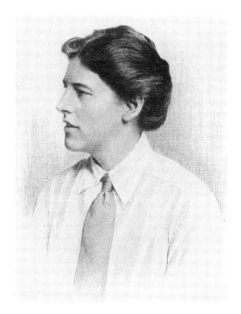

15.2 *Euphan Maxwell, FRCS. The first woman ophthalmic consultant in Ireland.*

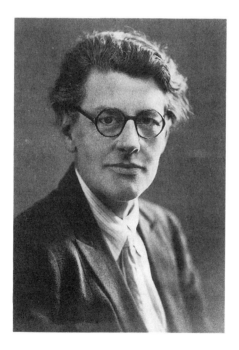

15.3 *Euphan Maxwell as senior surgeon.*

intelligent consensus a headline example of how to meet the twentieth century. Miss Maxwell's long and distinguished sojourn as surgeon to RVEEH extended into the memory of many still in practice; her moral impact on its public image will shortly become apparent.

For hospitals, as for most human enterprises, healthy finances determine the health of the individual. Initial euphoria arising from the decision to extend was no protection against demands for settlement of a bank overdraft now exceeding five thousand pounds. By September 1914 the Swanzy Memorial Fund had grown to a significant size and with trustees' permission it was agreed that its interest might be used as a small offset against the loan.

Even so, this barely checked a leak which was constantly worsening. Being privileged to project forward in time, we become aware that by November 1916 the situation had grown so dire as to justify the finance committee in recommending the issue of a special appeal. Council was advised to make individual approaches for assistance to subscribers in arrears, to the Dublin and Wicklow County Councils and to the parish priests of Ireland. Closure of the hospital in whole or in part would be the alternative unless funds were forthcoming. Sir Augustine Baker, a Council member, generously offered to pay for the appeal's publication in the daily papers. These various ploys were in preparation when the situation was transformed by an unforeseen bounty. Under the will of one E C Saunders a large legacy fell to be divided between certain named Dublin hospitals, RVEEH amongst them. This windfall proved to be worth more than £5000, and effectively ended the crisis.

Other bequests were more predictable but no less acceptable. On Arthur Benson's widow making a substantial donation in memory of her husband, Council proposed to respond by calling a new cataract ward after him, just as it intended to commemorate Swanzy by naming the West Wing in his honour. Regrettably these intentions were not implemented before larger issues intervened. When the resolves were made, even though fear of war was lively, it hardly seemed to threaten their accomplishment; yet before they could be realised the conflict had become reality. Six years later, the smoke cleared and the apocalyptic horsemen of war and disease no longer rode the earth, but the niceties of 1914 had been obliterated in the minds of the survivors.

If the diehard loyalty of the hospital to Crown and Establishment were not already clear to its supporters, the Great War was swift to put it to the proof. Two weeks after the declaration of war, Council approved a request from Miss Alice Reeves, the matron, to be allowed volunteer for active

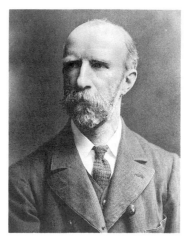

15.4 *Arthur H Benson. Coming from St Mark's, he was*
surgeon at RVEEH from 1897 to 1912. He became
eponymously celebrated for the description of
'Benson's Disease' (Asteroid Hyalitis).

service, appointing a senior sister as acting matron during her absence. Miss Reeves was a lady of forceful personality, which was ultimately to merit her high honours; her further career in RVEEH will be considered in due course. Her wartime activities culminated in appointment as senior sister in the King George V Military Hospital, a Red Cross establishment of 1650 beds, near London. For reasons unstated she did not persevere in this post, returning to RVEEH after an absence of five months.

Thereafter war items followed thick and fast in the minutes of Council business. An allocation of ten beds for military cases was agreed in September 1914, and a month later Dr James Beckett, just appointed as honorary anaesthetist to the hospital, gave notice that having accepted a position under the Red Cross he was compelled temporarily to relinquish his duties. Barely nine months in office, he trusted that Council would allow him resume work on his return. (This Beckett, namesake and nephew to the builder who had arbitrated with the Goods, was by that time uncle to the eight-year-old Samuel, the future playwright.) Among the consultant staff, temporary severance for army service was also sought and obtained by T O Graham ('Togo'), who was to win the Military Cross before his return, and also by Euphan Maxwell, who gathered the material for her second Montgomery Lecture during a sojourn on active service in Malta.

In January of 1914, the remuneration of house-surgeons had been adjusted to a complicated sliding scale allowing £40 p.a. for the first quarter, increasing thereafter by £10 a quarter up to a maximum of £70 a year. By the middle of 1915 there was such difficulty in getting house-surgeons, that for a short time resident students were employed, with remuneration of £2 a month and board and residence provided. When later a house-surgeon again became available he was offered a bonus of ten shillings a week on the regular salary, because of extra work arising from a solo appointment.

Wartime changes inevitably touched the hospital. The Scottish-born P W Maxwell died soon after his son was killed in action in 1916, and his daughter Euphan, already in the Royal Army Medical Corps and now abruptly deprived of her menfolk, returned to RVEEH, where for several decades she displayed a distinctive aura of her own.

The Euphan Maxwell who defines a period in RVEEH history was a slight figure with greying hair, a deep voice, and tweed coat and skirt which, blending with a striding gait, lent to the whole more than a hint of military determination. Possibly to accentuate her army experience she invariably wore a necktie, complementing that steady gaze and directness of manner which would have been at home in any Officers' Mess from Aldershot to India. Under these appearances, unique as any sketched by Dickens or Kipling, there lay a personality respected by all, and beloved by many for the forthright honesty of her nature. Trusty colleague and loyal friend, never seeking to dissemble the British origin which she carried as an article of faith, she yet accepted the principles of those around her as a fact of life, and was the epitome of a Christian gentlewoman.

It was impossible that an individual so positive could fail to impart a character to her surroundings. So was it that she set her stamp upon an era of the hospital's existence, imparting an aura of 'far-off things and battles long ago'. By succeeding Story as ophthalmologist to the Adelaide Hospital, through this appointment she presented in her own person the direct lineal descendant of both of the original joint senior surgeons of RVEEH. Those privileged to have known and worked with her, among them the present writer, may be permitted the fancy that in that contact they brushed the skirts of history.

Of the many intimations of future change occurring during the Great War period, there were naturally none more prophetic than the events of Easter 1916. Matron's report on them, incorporated in the Council minutes for May of that year, runs as follows:

> On Tuesday April 25th at 6.00 a.m. a soldier came in having been shot through the legs in Leeson St. On Thursday April 27th there were 30 empty beds here, and hearing that the Royal City of Dublin

Hospital was overcrowded, I told Dr Stoney we could take some patients. 42 soldiers were immediately sent over, 13 of them convalescents and the remainder Sherwood Foresters who had come in the night before, some only suffering from shock, but three or four with fairly serious wounds. Three more soldiers came here direct, making a total of 46 soldiers, and 116 patients all told, in hospital.

On May 5th we were asked to take 7 civilians who had been injured during the riots and treated at 40 Merrion Square, as that temporary hospital was being closed.

Very great difficulty was experienced for several days in getting sufficient food. Milk and meat came regularly, but it was impossible to get sugar or butter, and for two days the bread van failed to come; however by sending a messenger to the Castle we were able to get enough. The diet was considerably restricted for 5 or 6 days, but I do not think anybody was hungry. Dr T E Gordon very kindly looked after and operated on any case that required it and Dr Edward Watson took X-Ray photographs as needed, as it was impossible to get in touch with Dr Houghton. The neighbours kindly lent beds and offered sleeping accommodation for any soldiers who were able to be up and about. Several shots were fired into the sanitary block at the east end of the Hospital, and one into the out-patients department, but no one was injured.

15 of the soldiers were discharged on May 10th fit for duty, 16 transferred to King George V Hospital on May 13th and 12 more we expect to send away this week. There was a great deal of shooting and sniping all around this locality almost all the time, which made it most dangerous for anyone to come or go from here.

At the May meeting which received this report Council passed a vote of thanks to all friends who had assisted during a difficult time, as also to the hospital staff, with special mention of Miss Reeves the matron, and the registrar, Mr Howell. No reference was made at the time to the mysterious disappearance from the hospital practice of Dr Kathleen Lynn, who had been appointed clinical assistant since 1910. It was August before Council proceedings included the following minute: 'The medical board begs to draw the Council's attention to the fact that, since the recent rebellion Dr Kathleen Lynn had not attended the Hospital. She had neither applied for leave, sent in her resignation nor offered any explanation for her absence.' Owing to a small attendance, the matter was left over until the following meeting. By then a letter had been received from Dr Lynn, informing

Council she had returned to Dublin and was willing to resume work at the hospital if desired. Council's response was that owing to her prolonged absence other arrangements had been made and that her services as clinical assistant were no longer required. The corresponding vacancy was filled by the appointment of Dr Georgiana Prosser for one year.

Behind the bare factual record there lies a vignette of history fully described by Hazel P Smith in the *Dublin Historical Record* of March 1977 and sympathetically annotated in Dr David Mitchell's history of the Adelaide Hospital, both of which sources are acknowledged.

Kathleen Lynn was a daughter of the manse, her father having been rector of Cong in County Mayo. On her mother's side she was distantly related to Constance Gore-Booth, later Countess Markievicz. Born in the aftermath of the Famine, through a western childhood she is credited with that early awareness of social inequality which fired her with the aspiration to right it. In 1895 she enrolled as a student at the Adelaide Hospital, where she gained various prizes during the five years before graduating MB, B Ch at the Royal University, predecessor of the National University of Ireland – she had not followed the courses at Trinity since Dublin University did not accept women until 1903. Subsequent experience in Sir Patrick Dun's, the Rotunda, and RVEEH was followed by post-graduate work in the United States, after which she returned home, obtained her FRCSI in 1909 (only the tenth woman to do so) and, gaining lustre from her appointment at RVEEH, commenced practice in Rathmines as an eyespecialist.

So far, so good. But behind the always-caring practitioner there stood an individual far ahead of her time, whose social consciousness embraced not only women's suffrage, but also the political emancipation of the Irish people. She was particularly sensitive to the needs of women and children in those needy times. In these views she was influenced by her cousin Constance Markievicz and by Helena Moloney, secretary of the Women Workers Union of Ireland, through whom she became engaged in medical assistance to the stricken families of workers during the lock-out of 1913. From this it was but a step to joining the medical corps of the Citizen Army, of which she was soon made chief medical officer by James Connolly, its commandant.

This then was the background leading to Dr Lynn's protracted absence from hospital from Easter 1916 onwards. On that Easter Monday, she had reported at the College of Surgeons to her superior officer, Countess Markievicz, who drove her to the vicinity of Dublin Castle, where heavy casualties were expected. There, with other insurgents, she had secured entry to the City Hall, where she set up an improvised casualty clearing station, and where after the garrison commander had been killed it eventually fell to her as senior surviving officer, to make the surrender.

The description now mounted at the site dramatically portrays the scene, the soldiers rushing into the darkness of the central hall with an officer shouting, 'Anyone here? Speak or I'll shoot.' 'Dr Kathleen Lynn then stepped out of the shadows into the moonlight and surrendered the garrison.' She was arrested and imprisoned for a time, but was released before long, although the presence of a revolver alongside first-aid supplies in her medical bag made clear that in extremity her role could have been combatant as well as humanitarian.

From today's perspective this exploit can be squarely viewed as the adventure of an idealist. But from the then Establishment standpoint, the fervently loyalist authority of RVEEH must have shrunk from it with incredulous horror. In such circumstances the restrained reference in the minutes is laudably objective.

Dr Lynn resumed private practice and, dauntless woman that she was, soon found another cause to which she devoted the nearly forty years of professional life remaining to her. With her friend Madeline Ffrench Mullen, she set up the much-needed facility, St Ultan's Hospital. Initially for infants only, it was the first in Ireland – and possibly in these islands – to be dedicated to this age-group. Entirely staffed by women and subsisting largely on love, the foundation survived until 1980. Kathleen Lynn died in 1955, her funeral becoming a featured republican occasion, with three volleys fired over her grave. Upon this her biographer Hazel Smith commented: 'It is doubtful if this would have pleased Kathleen, the healer and helper, who grieved because the Christian Church was not pacifist.'

Meanwhile war or no war, the daily round in RVEEH went on, and with it the monthly records of wartime administration, today a useful archive. They ranged from such trivia as coping with the neighbours' objections to a smoke nuisance caused by the hospital furnace, to expensive necessities like the urgent need of re-painting if the building's fabric were not to decay. A continual rise in the price of commodities was balanced by problems of staffing, as when Matron could not get a new cook for less than £25 a year, while a gardener came to £1 a week, for which however he was also available to clean the windows.

Nursing matters had now gained an importance reflected in their regular discussion in Council business. Social legislation and the profession's enhanced prominence due to the high profile of its wartime activities had produced a manifest increase in its dignity and importance. Many decades were to elapse before it would be adopted as a faculty by RCSI, but when that day came RVEEH would be there to provide the initiative.

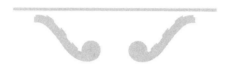

16

FROM SEED TO FRUIT IN
OPHTHALMIC NURSING

Prior to Florence Nightingale's establishment of nursing as a profession, skilled bed-care of the sick was largely the province of dedicated nuns, originators of the rank of 'Sister'. Such was the demand for general care that even for these religious, no formalised training seems to have existed for nursing of the special senses. This explains why early reports of St Mark's contain no reference to professional nursing care, since those going by the name of nurse were little more than orderlies capable of simple domestic duties.

In Wilde's annual reports it was 1857 before the nurse's role was mentioned. Indicating that both the consulting physician and surgeon were appointed by the Governors, the report went on: 'The Resident Assistant Surgeon and the Cupper, together with the Nurses, Porters and other Officers of the Institution, are engaged by and remain under the control of the Surgeon; for each of these appointments there are specific laws and rules to which the holders must be amenable.'

The rules for the nurse provided that she was to sleep in the female ward, receive the same diet as the patients, with named supplements, and to have a bonus of one shilling a week besides her wages. She was to leave immediately on being so required by the surgeon, in which case she would be paid a week's wages on top of any pay outstanding. Her duties included the washing of towels and linen, maintenance of cleanliness, and accountability for items of hospital property under her care. It was her responsibility to see that no patient left the hospital without medical permission, neglect of such duty being liable to a maximum fine of one shilling.

It is evident that in 1857 the role of the 'nurse' in St Mark's was essentially that of a superior washerwoman with some extra duties, not involving a ministry of patients or technical knowledge of any sort. The dating of the report is crucial to our comprehension, being just one year after Florence Nightingale had returned from Scutari; by this time she was in London, embarked on her crusade for formal training of a true generation of nurses at St Thomas' and King's College Hospitals. Although as for centuries before, surgery at the time was a recognised art with its modified successes, there still lacked three years before Lister would revolutionise its practice by his introduction of antisepsis.

Wilde's reports, both in style and content, invariably made good reading. His annual analysis and statistical classification of diseases vied with a yearly account of the hospital's steady progress as a teaching centre, and there can be no doubt of his extreme pride in this. But even as every eye has its blind spot, for him the vaunted increase in ophthalmic knowledge among students and young doctors seems to have posed no collateral sense of need for educated carers. While being of course a man of his time, the time itself was one when fresh knowledge percolated slowly. As a result, while news of the Nightingale and Lister revolutions would have reached him as one rich indeed in achievement, he was by then already approaching old age.

The 1877 report gave striking proof of change. It will be remembered that Wilde had died the year before, to be succeeded by his natural son Henry Wilson, and that in tragic turn the latter had died within the year. Besides recording his death, the report for 1877 therefore dealt also with Wilson's one year in office. Significantly, the account of this carried news of an advance which of itself would distinguish his governance as effecting a unique watershed in patient care. The record ran: 'A beneficial change has been made in the nursing department and the post of Matron established, the first appointment being that of Mrs Sarah Galvan who has given entire satisfaction.'

This beginning, made as the nineteenth century entered its last quarter, was not to be without setbacks. By the following year not only had the satisfactory Mrs Galvan been replaced by a Miss Molony, but following London practice, the job description itself was changed to that of lady superintendent. The Board expressed itself as well satisfied with its second incumbent, stating that since the appointment many valuable improvements had been made in internal management of the hospital.

Alas for human endeavour! Yet another year and Miss Molony too had departed, because of 'her refusal to engage a trained nurse as directed by the Board of Governors'. Her successor, Miss Beresford, initially non-resident, was described as having a large and varied superintendent experience in Dublin and London. Unlike Miss Molony, she did not scorn having a trained nurse under her direction and earned acknowledgement by name and office on the report's title page.

This appointment occurred in 1879. A patient of the time left a written eulogy of his month's stay in St Mark's for cataract removal. Entitled 'A voice from St Mark's – how I recovered my eyesight', and published in the *Kilkenny Moderator*, it is annotated in Story's writing as the work of one Mr Innes, a friend of Charles Lever the novelist. Describing the operation the cured patient wrote: 'The performers in this little drama were Dr Story in chief, Dr Beattie assisting, a friendly doctor held the pulse, and the handsome Fanny Campbell, chief hospital nurse, was also in attendance. Two doctors and a few medical students formed the spectators. Carbolic spray was used on the occasion.' For all his affliction of sight, Mr Innes was obviously not immune to the charms of a pretty girl.

Miss Beresford may be seen as the first serious occupant of the matron's post, which in 1883 became a resident one. When she left, the Board gave her a testimonial in appreciation of the improved nursing system she had instituted. With her successor, Miss Wall, trained at Addenbrooke's Hospital in Cambridge, we project into this century, as she endured to become one of the two joint matrons at the amalgamation.

Meanwhile at the National the topic of nursing was not mentioned until 1880, when removal to Molesworth Street evoked reference to a matron's apartments and ample accommodation for nurses. Two years later the Governors abolished the system of board wages and resolved that in future the matron, nurses and servants would be boarded by the hospital. Up to this, nursing staff had apparently been recruited from an agency, the Holles St Nurses Institution, and it was Swanzy who drew the Board's attention to the advantage of having a permanent nurse instead of the agency arrangement of quarterly rotation. His suggestion would cost an additional £10 a year, but as two 'Friends' (i.e. Quakers) had offered to give that amount annually for this very purpose, the Board decided to deal accordingly with the agency.

In that year of 1882, a Miss Trench wrote to inform the Board that her institution could no longer abide by a previous agreement to supply a probationer nurse without payment. £10 a year was now asked for her services, in addition to the £20 being paid for the matron. The latter salary was in turn revised when on second thoughts the agency reckoned, in view of the 'very superior nurse' required as matron, the sum agreed would put it to a loss in the current year; it proposed raising the amount to £30 in years following. At this the Board volunteered to pay the going rate immediately rather than see the Institute out of pocket. Such courteous example of *noblesse oblige* offers a miniature reflection of the voluntary hospital ethos, honourable behaviour being but second nature to the Governors.

At the National the first named matron was Miss Andrews, noticed in 1882 when installation of a fireplace in her sittingroom called attention to her establishment. The earliest duty devolving on her was a long way removed from nursing, the Board having directed her to arrange that henceforth the cook, alone among the servants, should have an allowance of porter.

By the time of her resignation in 1883 the Board had decided to control its own destiny in future, by means of direct appointment, its choice for the post being a Miss Huxley. Between the lines one can read that this move caused offence to the nursing agency, which soon afterwards abruptly withdrew its probationer so that the Board's earlier gentility was ill-rewarded. The hospital had further upset the established order by deciding to pay an enhanced salary to the matron. The National's complete emancipation from nursing dependence came early in 1884, when decisions were made both to increase the nurse's salary to £14 a year and to provide complete board and lodging for her as soon as convenient. This elimination of the middleman saw the achievement of nursing autonomy.

Meanwhile the physical conditions of accommodation were slowly being improved. Starting with matron acquiring her own quarters, little by little advances in her status are recorded, by a rise of salary here, a writing table there, now a request for leave granted 'with pleasure', next a carpet for her sittingroom. The choice of Miss Huxley, trained in Barts, had been an excellent one, but destiny beckoned and her outstanding ability determined a swift flitting to Sir Patrick Dun's, where in her term as matron she founded a training school and became the pioneer of modern nursing in Dublin. Not surprisingly, the keen judgement of its selectors determined that the National retained few of its early matrons for more than a year. It took Miss Gertrude Knight, who came from the Radcliffe Infirmary in

Oxford and stayed three years at the National, to make what may be seen as a definitive impact on it.

Her advent had evoked a mixed reaction. She had barely assumed office when in November 1885 the Board was moved to complain of increased expenditure on meat for the previous month. Enquiry showed that this was due to her discontinuing the serving of an oxhead dinner once a week; she had replaced it with ordinary meat instead. The Board instructed the oxhead dinner to be resumed but that it be made as palatable as possible. Soon after, when cook's wages were raised to 11/8d a month it was hinted that her attention should be drawn to the cooking of the oxheads.

Miss Knight stayed for three and a half years, finally leaving to become matron of the Adelaide. Years later this departure on promotion would be repeated in the case of Miss Reeves who, Adelaide-trained, moved to become matron of Dr Steevens' Hospital. The progression of each of these ladies to a major general hospital reflected how service in RVEEH was seen to add lustre to those who worked there. On recognising the reason for Miss Knight's 'extravagance' in preferring a superior diet for her patients, the Board's esteem for her grew rapidly, with annual acknowledgement of her dedicated attention. The flavour of her positive personality also infuses the Board's warm thanks for the 'very beautiful' oil painting she executed for the men's day room. Her resignation was much regretted; on departure her virtues were lauded as constancy, attention, courtesy and tact.

Her successor, Miss Lee, was the last matron of the National as a separate entity, since Miss Hosford, who followed, was responsible to successive authorities before and after amalgamation. There is no account of special sense issues encountered by Miss Lee, but while at the National she promoted nursing education, drawing up the syllabus for a Nursing Science course she mounted there in 1894. The degree of skill expected of ophthalmic nurses at that time remains uncertain, though Miss Lee surely had ambitions for her course, described in the *Freeman's Journal* as 'advanced teaching for nurses'.

However, the records make it seem likely that for long the National enjoyed the services of only a single staff nurse, named in 1886 as Nurse Walsh. Her growing importance is apparent from frequent salary increases grudgingly granted by the Board, in contrast with its earlier largesse to the agency. For instance, when in 1889 it was agreed to award her a raise of £2, making a total salary of £20 a year, the minute sternly defined it as being final. Nevertheless, in 1893 her salary was increased to £25, and two years later rose to £30 at matron's specific request. The inference is that skill born of experience had made her first of the long line of staff nurses later to be the pride of RVEEH.

It has been explained how from 1897 to 1904 the new hospital abode in the two branches of St Mark's and the National, with their respective lady superintendents sharing joint supremacy over nursing in RVEEH. The dual system persisted until Miss Wall's retirement in 1903, after which, in a single hospital with unitary control, the era of twentieth-century nursing can fairly be said to have begun. 1904, inaugural year of the RVEEH building, offers a moment in time when the need of a modern nursing system can be seen as casting its shadow forward. The hospital's subsequent history was to determine evolution of ophthalmic nursing as a specialised department in itself.

First however, the impact of amalgamation has to be examined. Even though the hospital would be under two roofs for a further seven years, combination of the two units as a corporate entity in 1897 gave an automatic fillip to the nursing. The existence of two lady superintendents (later called matrons) was a clear invitation for them to interact in moulding something new out of a now common background. Sure enough, there arose before long a problem calculated to exercise the best efforts not only of themselves but of Council also. Following accidental death of an in-patient in 1899, the question arose as to whether there existed a need for night nursing of eye patients. The inquest had raised legal and ethical questions troublesome to the collective conscience of Council. These were lucidly set out in an official letter signed by Swanzy as secretary and addressed to the hospital solicitors.

It was only after Senior Counsel's opinion had been taken that scruples arose as to whether all aspects of the case had been covered. Swanzy wrote: 'The point made by Mr Brady who represented the relations at the inquest, and presumably the point which would be mainly relied on before a judge and jury, is the following: The managers of the hospital provide no regular night nurse to attend upon the patients as they ought to do, and as is done in other hospitals. Had a night nurse been in attendance, the accident would not have occurred. The hospital authorities do not represent the hall porter as having been in the ward for the purpose of looking after the patients. Consequently the Council of the hospital is liable for the accident. The Hospital authorities in reply would say: This is an eye hospital. The patients have diseases of their eyes, but otherwise are in good health, and need no night nurse. They sleep soundly all night. When occasionally a patient is seriously ill otherwise than as regards his eyes, a night nurse is got in, as also in certain cases of eye diseases. The charge that the hospital authorities ought to have had a night nurse in attendance is the point which I do not feel sure as being covered by Counsel's opinion.'

This reasoned sequence of argument exemplifies Swanzy's analytical approach. As a result of this heart-searching, in August 1899 a circular letter was issued from the registrar to various eye hospitals in the UK, mostly those with one hundred beds or over, including Moorfields and the Royal Eye in London, and also eye hospitals in Birmingham, Manchester, Liverpool and Glasgow. Stating merely that the provision of night nurses in ophthalmic hospitals had been questioned in Dublin, on behalf of Council it sought information as to local use of night nurses in these centres. Was a night nurse on duty regularly? – and if so, what was the nurse/bed ratio? Did the local management regard a night nurse in ophthalmic hospitals as being necessary on a regular basis? – the custom in Dublin having been to employ such assistance only in exceptional circumstances.

No reply to this circular has come to light. It is nevertheless of peculiar interest in dating the evolving history of ophthalmic nursing. Up to this Dublin's eye hospitals had been small if respected units beside the several larger ones in Britain. Within five years RVEEH was to emerge as certainly the newest, and also one of the largest establishments in these islands. The evidence that only so recently did night nursing of ophthalmic cases become a moral imperative is itself a commentary on both social and technical developments occurring this century.

As to staff numbers and salary it appears that prior to 1900 the nursing establishment of the newly incorporated hospital was neither large nor highly organised. The wording of a minute of 1898 mentioning 'the present staff nurse of the National branch' suggests there was only one such appointment in the National. An authorised replacement for her was to be 'fully competent' at a salary not to exceed £30 a year. Unless in the unlikely event of a differential salary existing between the two branches, it seems to have been unnecessary to approach even this limit, since two years later a rise of £2 brought the St Mark's staff nurse's salary up to £27 per annum.

The first reference to junior nurses occurs in 1904 when opening of the fine RVEEH building was seen to add prestige to the fact of working there. Early that year the chairman of Sir Patrick Dun's wrote to ask that the system of instructing probationer nurses should be continued, as management thought the special training to be of great advantage to the nurses. In agreeing the continuation, RVEEH stipulated that the two-monthly tour of duty be increased by a month, and that the probationers presented should be of not less than one year's standing, conditions which were immediately accepted by the other side. Between the lines, it is fairly clear that a previous arrangement existed with Sir Patrick Dun's; in practice the presence of these young probationers in RVEEH, albeit for a short term and in training, would have helped in providing accessory labour at little cost to the hospital.

The system of dual matronship ended in 1903 with the retirement of Miss Wall. First appointed to St Mark's in 1884, she was the last of the old-style matrons, filling a role that was probably more domestic than professional. Her prolonged service had earned her both smiles and frowns from the Council, as exemplified in one letter praising her efficiency in reducing dietary costs by a penny farthing a day, or in another exhorting economy because of a gas bill for £45 covering a six-month period. Her honourable retirement cleared the way for the opening of the new building under the unitary rule of Miss Hosford.

The latter's ten years of service to RVEEH ended in 1908 when she left to get married; thus, by inference, she brought a young and energetic presence to the launching of the new institution. Coming as she did, from the National, previous collaboration with Swanzy would have generated in each a mutual respect for the other. The excellent job she did in putting the new hospital into working order was acknowledged in a handsome tribute from Council on her departure, when amid a clutch of clichés special thanks were offered for 'the efficient manner in which she organised the internal affairs of the hospital, on occupation of the present buildings in 1904, when the chief burden of this arrangement fell on her'. A contemporary photograph of the nursing staff shows it to have comprised at least twelve persons including the matron.

When Miss Hosford resigned in 1908 the prestige of the hospital was such that no fewer than forty-four applicants applied to succeed her. The choice fell on Miss Alice Reeves, whose career has earlier been touched upon. The daughter of a clergyman and granddaughter of a former president of the Royal Irish Academy, before coming to RVEEH she had trained and worked at the Adelaide, surely a bonus in establishing relations with Swanzy. In her person sterling character was balanced by versatility, as when on the registrar's falling ill in 1912 she and another ascendant star, Winifred Jackson, then a junior clerk, were jointly charged with keeping the accounts during his absence. Again, while observing her war service to have been honoured with the major decoration of the Royal Red Cross, she loses no dignity in the tale of her seeking permission to erect a henhouse in hospital grounds at her own expense. Rather the contrary, since the reason for this apparent eccentricity was directed to the common good, enabling experiments in intensive egg production during dire days of rationing.

Including wartime wanderings, Miss Reeves' association with RVEEH lasted eleven years before her departure in 1918 to become matron of Dr Steevens' Hospital. She left on RVEEH the imprint of disciplined nursing it has borne ever since. The career of this born achiever, twice a distinguished matron, attracted public notice in 1922 when she brought the newly formed Irish Free State into the International Council of Nurses, and in 1925 through her influential role in framing rules for the new General Nursing Council of Ireland (now An Bord Altranais). It culminated in 1947 when she was awarded the honorary degree of MA from Trinity College Dublin.

She was succeeded by Miss E M Power, who had been successively theatre sister and acting matron during Miss Reeves' wartime absence. Her reign lasted from 1918 to 1931; while producing no spectacular nursing changes, it marked a time of further social evolution, including the end of the Great War quickly followed by the foundation of the Free State. Her special achievement lay in keeping nursing services on an even keel during a difficult time in history, no mean feat in view of this being the decade which saw the original plan for the hospital finally completed. She well played the role of consolidator. She lived for some thirty years after retirement, and her fund-raising ploy in amassing a mile of sixpences lingers in reminder of her zeal.

It was during this period there occurred the unusual case of Miss Mary Connolly. A staff sister under Miss Power, she showed such aptitude for ophthalmology as to encourage her to embark upon a career change. Undaunted by the many consequent problems, she qualified in medicine and later ophthalmology, ending up on the surgical staff of the hospital she had entered as a nurse.

With Miss Allen, who followed Miss Power in 1931, we enter the modern era. It is now sixty years since she assumed office, a period when the nursing destinies of RVEEH have been under the care of no more than three matrons, the Misses Allen, Prunty and Fitzsimons. Whether clinically, administratively, or in the quality of care, all have added distinction to the office, a process which continues today, Miss Fitzsimons having attained Council membership on personality alone, independent of rank.

In the overall nursing scene other names, some alas of those no longer living, call for recognition as part of the fibre of RVEEH in their time.

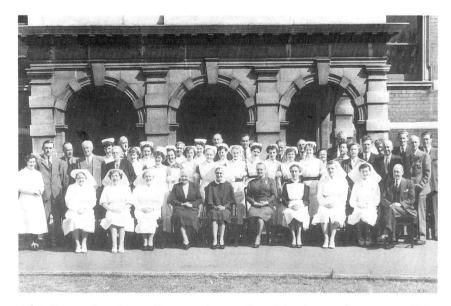

16.1 *Group of nursing staff seen on the occasion of the change of matrons in 1957. Sitting: Dr M O'Connell, Sr May Moloney, Sr Nancy Barry, Sr Lucy Kelleher, Miss E M Allen, Miss Mary Prunty, Miss M F Crowley, Sr K Lennon, Sr D McBrien, Mr P D Piel.*

Sisters Lucy Kelleher and May Moloney laboured for forty-six and forty-two years respectively, known and respected by generations of doctors and patients as pillars of the institution. During the expanding decades of the sixties and seventies, Miss Mary Dunford as Eye Theatre sister brought calm and competence to bear on the many crises of those changeful years. Sister Nora Quade served a thirty-nine year tour of duty before quitting the Casualty Department to enter on the honourable retirement she now enjoys.

However, the name most prominent in the public eye was that of Miss Mary Frances Crowley, whose pioneer work in the field of ophthalmic nurse training made a landmark for the profession in Ireland. A native of County Cork, she first came to prominence soon after World War II, on being granted leave of absence from RVEEH to engage in post-war relief work in Europe. Posted to St Lo in Normandy, she there acted as matron in the temporary hospital set up by the Irish Red Cross Society. On completion of her mission she was decorated by the French Government with a Medal of Gratitude before returning to Ireland and resuming her dual office as assistant matron and sister tutor.

In 1945 RVEEH had been recognised for nurse training by the Irish

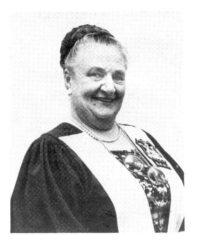

16.2 *Mary Frances Crowley, who founded the School of*
Nursing at RVEEH and became the first dean of the
Faculty of Nursing at RCSI.

General Nursing Council, with affiliation to three general hospitals, Sir Patrick Dun's, Dr Steevens' and the Meath. Expanded in 1947, by 1949 the teaching activity was ripe for recognition as the Ophthalmic Nurse Training School, devised and conducted by Miss Crowley as a post-graduate educational opportunity for qualified nurses. The final step came in 1951 with the introduction of a standardised Diploma in Ophthalmic Nursing, confined to registered nurses and having RVEEH as the course centre for Ireland. It provided a year of training, and included arrangements whereby student staff nurses were admitted to undergraduate lectures in ophthalmology at UCD.

In this way did ophthalmic nursing come of age as a specialised form of patient care, with Mary Frances Crowley as unquestioned prime mover in a development conferring prestige on both profession and hospital. Her part in this was suitably recognised by her appointment as first dean of RCSI's Faculty of Nursing on its foundation in 1974. Other distinctions in a rich career of accomplishment included that of examiner to the Ophthalmic Nursing Board in England and presidency of the Academic Society of Nurse Tutors. Miss Crowley died in 1990, having been associated with RVEEH almost to the last day of her life. Through her enduring bequest of its training school for ophthalmic nursing she made it her lasting debtor.

17

LIFE AFTER SWANZY

Forty years after Wilde's demise, the passing of Sir Henry Swanzy saw an end to the hospital's Heroic Age. Between them, these two had sustained more than seventy years of continuous institutional activity; at the date of Swanzy's death in 1913 there lacked only a single year to complete the cycle of a century since Ryall's pioneering venture. Since that distant foundation, Irish ophthalmology had enjoyed rare good fortune in successively raising up two such gigantic figures, standing back to back as it were, during its growth to maturity.

In swift succession to Sir Henry's disappearance from the scene came a series of epochal changes, in the form of war, revolution and the foundation of a new State, things such as fully justified the epitome of Yeats: 'Changed, changed, utterly changed; a terrible beauty is born.' The concatenation of all these factors within the space of less than ten years had the effect of standing the established order on its head, thereby requiring of any institution an exceptional degree of stability merely to secure survival. In this RVEEH was not to be found wanting, and the measure of its guiding principles would soon be seen in a disciplined adaptation to the new order.

To a foundation so firmly grounded on loyalty to the Crown and its institutions, the 1922 establishment of a national Government in Dublin

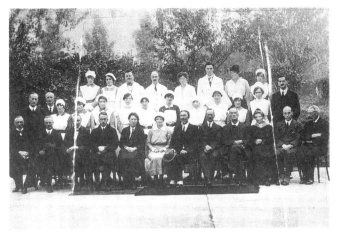

17.1 *Staff group, c.1922*

can hardly have come as a welcome development. It says much for the proper conduct of Council affairs, that whatever the affront sustained in personal feelings, never do the minutes betray the slightest hint of ruffled sensibilities, and that hospital business continued exactly as before. The underlying resilience proving the hospital's capacity to survive was nowhere better seen than in the report for 1923 and the AGM at which it was presented.

Here was an occasion where inclination and expediency combined. The premier dignitary of the newly formed Irish Free State was the Governor General, who in the person of the celebrated Tim Healy KC, now occupied the Viceregal Lodge. Following the well-tried formula of identification with the Establishment, Council invited him to attend and address the meeting. A better choice could hardly have been made. On the one hand he bore the lustre of a Crown-approved appointment, on the other this erstwhile associate of Parnell, speaking in the accent of West Cork, was as Irish as the shamrock. Thus, equipped to meet any occasion, he was also a skilful barrister endowed with the gift of the gab.

He struck the right note immediately. Having avowed as his aim the encouragement of subscriptions, he launched into a topical reminiscence, recalling how in 1869 he had come up from his native Bantry to attend Sir William Wilde at St Mark's in Lincoln Place. Citing this as evidence that the hospital was no mere metropolitan asset but a national one also, he went on to eulogise Wilde, both for medical skill and renown as archaeologist and historian. Fully aware of the loyalist fires still burning in his audience, the wily advocate wheedled its attention with a story involving Wilde and

Queen Victoria, telling how the monarch had engaged the famous oculist to care for the eyes of Princess Beatrice, her youngest daughter, whom he had cured. It can not have failed in reassuring its hearers that the new regime had such a civil recollection of the old.

The peroration of this clever speech combined a summary of its themes with a percipient glance at the future. In this hospital he saw himself as speaking to the common humanity of all creeds and classes. Reflecting on the special senses as being among the most delicate and wonderful attributes of the human race, he surmised that thanks to the marvellous acoustic inventions of the day there was new hope that the senses would benefit, since it was now possible to hear from hundreds of miles what ten years ago could not be heard a hundred yards away.

Long before marvels like microsurgery and the hearing-aid were invented, this speech showed remarkable foresight that technology would rule the future. In a sense it also adumbrated a revised charter for revised circumstances, in other words that creed and class would in time be supplanted by the common name of Irishman. To an audience containing many who must have been sceptical of the new State, it showed that regardless of whether the accent was that of west Britain or west Cork, authority still existed. In taking the bull by the horns and referring to the pluralist aspect of the hospital he directed a long look forward to the ecumenical dialogue it would ultimately enjoy. If Swanzy's death had marked the watershed between nineteenth and twentieth centuries, then the coming of independence saw another frontier defined in quiet attainment of an interdenominational hospital based on Christian principles.

It was in 1924 that the name of Harvey Lewis first appeared in the minutes. This was the name to be given to the West Wing of RVEEH, which would complete Swanzy's vision, despite the fact that previously there had been no known connection between the Harvey Lewis family and the hospital.

John Harvey Lewis was a one-time MP and high sheriff for County Kildare. His widow, Jane Isabella, directed in her will that from the settlement of her estate a sum of £80,000 be used to build and endow in Dublin 'the Harvey Lewis Memorial Hospital' in memory of her husband. She died in 1904, but for a variety of reasons the will was still unsettled by 1925, when only £22,000 of the intended sum remained for the proposed hospital. This was clearly not enough, so it fell to the courts to assign the bequest. Dublin's hospitals were invited to submit applications, and twenty-four of them responded. Bearing in mind that the original intention of the will was to build a new hospital, the court ruled that completion of the Royal Victoria Eye and Ear Hospital most nearly matched the wishes of Mrs Harvey Lewis since it would ensure that the entire legacy was spent on a single project. It was not the court's business to deal with parentheses: with a depleted estate there could be no reference to the total impossibility of meeting the will's specific instruction to invest the residue of estate towards upkeep and maintenance of the hospital. The lack of this endowment was to prove a grave handicap in the future.

By this roundabout means, Swanzy's vision at last came within sight of completion. The immediate jubilation would be succeeded by sobering considerations, such as wastage through costs amounting to nearly one third of the remaining legacy, as well as the thousand details of equipment. But in March 1925 all was well, and the AGM following soon after the judgment was adorned with such a panel of speakers as showed how truly it is said that 'nothing succeeds like success'. There was the lord chief justice, the provost of Trinity College and governor of the Bank of Ireland, and the presidents of both the Colleges of Physicians and of Surgeons in Ireland. Many words were spoken by these grave persons, most of them to do with funding; of their remarks probably the most prescient came from the Rev J H Bernard, the provost of TCD. Foreseeing the impossibility of supporting an ever-increasing expenditure from voluntary subscriptions, the more so at a time when many moneyed people had left the country, he voiced the thought that perhaps it was time for the financing of such institutions by a general tax of some kind. Here was prophetic utterance: a small voice foretelling in 1925 something which would become the Department of Health's billion-pound budget of the nineties.

However, at the time of entering the second quarter of the century, when the entire country's annual budget came to less than thirty million pounds, the raising of funds for day-to-day expenses was still very much the business of Council. Besides heralding the hospital's new wing, the AGM of 1926 introduced a fresh character destined for future prominence on the hospital scene. Attending as an invited speaker, Gordon Campbell, Lord Glenavy, took the opportunity to conduct a sort of public audit of accounts presented to the meeting. Having long held senior rank as a civil servant, he was qualified to indicate possible lines of improvement, and to deplore the unfortunate necessity of using bequests for running expenses. This habit of command, helped no doubt by possession of a title, made so favourable an impression on Council that when in 1932 Sir George Roche died while in office, Lord Glenavy was to become his successor and commence a new era.

Meanwhile we are running ahead of time, with Sir George still hale and hearty. A prominent solicitor, and the only survivor of the original Council of RVEEH, he was highly desirous of seeing the building completed in his time. To a hospital so permanently short of beds, once the court award was made there was every reason to move smartly. Instead for some reason there intervened a delay unexplained in the archives. This added nine months to the interval between bestowal of the award and the appearance of plans, after which a further eight months passed before August 1926, when work started. By now Batchelor had retired and returned to his native country, being succeeded as hospital architect by Hicks, his junior. The builders of the new wing were H and J Martin, whose contract price of just under £14,000 was accepted, linked to a time schedule of sixty-five weeks.

As with any building work there were a few hitches, but none this time due to builders' intransigence. Their only deviation from plan occurred when a strike of brickworkers impeded the use of specified materials, leading to a proposed modification which was accepted. Council's difficulties lay elsewhere. No sooner was a firm of quantity surveyors engaged than a rival firm disputed the appointment, alleging existence of an agreement from 1900 giving them prior entitlement. This claim was successfully resisted as being time-expired. Finally, when the work was half completed, it became apparent that a momentous choice was necessary, with the emergence of a now-or-never situation. Was the building to stop at the second floor as budgeted, or was the façade to be made fully symmetrical by the addition of another storey with a Mansard roof? This was costed as amounting to an extra £1000; posterity must forever be debtor to a courageous Council which, rather than mutilate the architecture of a noble building, agreed to accept the extra burden.

Nevertheless it must have been with trepidation that the growing edifice was seen to approach completion. Before the work was six months in hand, it became necessary to seek an extra overdraft of £3000 from the bank, and when towards the end of 1927 construction work ended, funds for painting were so low that the architect offered to defray the cost of exterior painting himself. During that year, Council had been put to an exceptional expense arising from the will of the late Marquess of Ely, whose bequest to the hospital was subject to the life interest of his widow. This meant RVEEH would not benefit until her death, while an unusual clause required the hospital to contribute £100 towards the deceased's funeral expenses. At such a straitened time this was truly stressful, but in the light of expectations the charge had to be met in pious hope that the widow would not squander.

This haemorrhage from a body already anaemic possibly represented the nadir of RVEEH fortunes. Yet in spite of being so near to financial extinction, the hospital refused to lie down, surviving through the will of its officers to hold on. Though the now-completed West Wing had space for forty beds, it perforce remained unused for want of furnishing. Since there was no way to go but forward, it was decided to have a formal opening in the hope that creating an occasion would attract subscribers. The Rt Hon James MacNeill, then Governor General, was invited to perform the ceremony on 18 July 1928. Were it but known, the very instrument of ceremony, in the form of an ornamental gold key presented to him, had itself to be provided through the personal generosity of Sir George Roche, president of Council.

There was a mixed attitude among the several speakers on this quasi-festive occasion. Where the optimists rejoiced in the completed structure, the down-to-earth realists stressed Council's 'very considerable anxiety' at the financial state of the hospital. Though the number of patients admitted showed an increase of 400 on the previous year, the operating deficit for the year came to over £2000; and the absence of income from invested funds was especially noted.

All had been agreed that the canvassing of extra subscribers was essential, but a year later despite sustained pressure of admissions, the wing still stood idle. Thanks to the individual efforts of Mrs Christopher Murphy, wife of a Council member, one large ward had been substantially equipped, but eleven were still empty, and a special appeal was launched to raise the sum of about £1200 still required. The resulting surge of extra effort produced a crop of entertainments, tournaments and raffles as well as the more solid income of subscriptions. By March 1930 the final phase of the 1904 design was at last commissioned, adding some thirty extra beds to the establishment.

It appears necessary to give an explanatory coda to present-day users and friends of the hospital. Despite a large brass plate defining its provenance, by a quirk of usage the title of 'Harvey Lewis Wing' has become confined in practice to the suite of private and semi-private rooms housed in the north-west arm of the 'H' design of the hospital. It is only just to emphasise that the Harvey Lewis appellation embraces the entire western block of the building and that to the name of Harvey Lewis the institution owes not merely a private facility, but the fact of its completion.

18

CHANGES IN THE BACKGROUND

The death of Sir George Roche at the beginning of the thirties was a definitive event for the hospital. In his person he had seen completed the task initiated by a Council of which he was the sole survivor. His passing was therefore a clear marker between epochs. Behind lay the stately Victorian values, while in front was the brisker practice of the twentieth century, already shaping to be the era of the common man. To guide the hospital in this new age, there now came forward a doughty triad, comprising one man and two women, destined by force of character to occupy key positions for the next quarter-century.

Lord Glenavy has already been mentioned. Although he had not hitherto been a member, Council unanimously resolved to offer him its presidency on the death of Sir George Roche. He took up this position in February 1932, when as chance would have it, a new matron, Miss Ethel Allen, was barely two months in office. She would prove to be a rock of stability and common sense.

Complementing these two was Miss Winifred Jackson, whose steady rise through the ranks since her appointment in 1911 as dispensary clerk on a salary of twelve shillings a week had culminated in her becoming registrar in 1921. From the start of her employment, constant recurrence of her name in the records marked her out as one ever willing to serve wherever the situation demanded, and regular notes of Council's appreciation indicated how well her ability was recognised. Along with these gifts she brought an invaluable knowledge of hospital affairs, still lacking to her new colleagues at the top.

In the century's fourth decade, although the long gradient of fund-raising for construction had at last been surmounted, the perennial cash crisis remained. The financial constraints of the twenties having been common to all voluntary hospitals, and private charity being a limited resource, an evolving society had to devise new methods. Fresh schemes of raising and distributing funds were plainly necessary, and this was how in the early thirties, based on the model of the famous Calcutta Sweep, the idea of an Irish Hospitals Sweepstake was born.

Though its success is now a matter of history, the venture had its opponents; their objections were based on a principled opposition to gambling. Chief among them was the Adelaide Hospital, which conscientiously refused to abandon principle, even at the cost of exclusion from funds accessible to its peers. Although RVEEH had for long shared a common ethic with the Adelaide, in the present matter Council agonised for some time as to its correct attitude, eventually deciding that the sheer plight of the hospital demanded adherence to the Sweep as the only option; moreover, in a mixed Council the extremity of conscientious scruple was diluted. This may indeed have been the juncture unrecognised at the time, when RVEEH finally broke from the tradition of Crown and Establishment, allowing independence of judgement to prove it had an identity of its own.

To the present generation, accustomed to a weekly lottery, the dilemma may seem to have been doctrinaire. In the sixty years since the Sweep was launched the pressures of an entertainment industry has altered the public perception of gambling to a marked extent, not necessarily for the better. However, without being judgemental, today's thoughtful observer can afford to respect both the Adelaide's staunchness to its Protestant principles and the realistic reaction of RVEEH, whose bending to the gale almost certainly saved it from foundering.

Out of these manoeuvrings there came into existence two new institutions, the one rooted in private enterprise, the other a creature of the State. These were respectively, the family organisation set up by the celebrated Joe McGrath and known as Hospitals Trust, which ran the Sweep and raised the much-needed cash, and the Hospitals Commission, empowered by State to ensure the money's fair distribution. Despite their diverse origins these two were as complementary to one another as

Tweedledum and Tweedledee. Together, for several decades they formed for funding an effective bridge between the haphazard system of a time when it was entirely voluntary, and today's budgetary arrangement of massive dependence on the State.

And where, it may be asked, did the Department of Health feature in this scenario? For today's observer the astonishing answer is that sixty years ago, a Department of Health, as such, did not exist. The current personal and political importance of health delivery is due to technological developments then still in the womb of time. In those days, medical items needing adjudication came under jurisdiction of the Department of Local Government and Public Health, a twin appointment for a minister for whom there were as many votes in the state of county roads as in the waiting lists for cataracts, squints and tonsils, if indeed such lists existed. The setting up of the Hospitals Commission seems to have been this department's answer to the problem of its own split personality, ultimately to be solved by creation of a separate ministry.

In the growing apparatus of State therefore, for some decades the official link for hospitals lay more with the Commission than directly with 'the department', and a state of mutual understanding evolved into a reasonable working relationship. True, there was still invariably an annual deficit; true also there were still private subscribers, the oscillation of whose bounty was carefully watched, with life-membership of the hospital still a titbit for the generous. But while nobody would have admitted it, the haunted days of hand-to-mouth were receding, and a period had been reached when the budget shortfall of any one year could reasonably be expected to be made good by the Commission in the next. The Health Acts, with payment of doctors for work done, were still far in the future; equally so, with hindsight it is now possible to recognise that the career of the voluntary hospital as an entirely private charity had passed its zenith; and the advent of a State-funded service was only biding its time.

In such circumstances, some loss of dimension in the hospital's story is inevitable at this stage of its history. When Robert Louis Stevenson wrote that hopeful travelling is better than arrival, he predicated the controlled excitement that had invested the hospital for almost forty years. Now with building completed, the challenge accepted and victory won, the blush of achievement, unless nurtured, would cease to bloom. RVEEH had indeed arrived, but there remained the duty of conservation.

Since with the structure finished incentive was lost, it is hardly surprising that after the West Wing was raised, for some years Council records appear as something of a plateau, an ordered but featureless

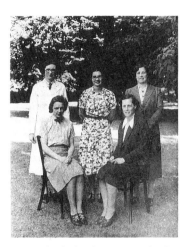

18.1 *Group showing the lady almoner and administrative staff in the 1930s. Seated, from left: Miss Earl, Miss McIntosh; Standing: Miss D Connor (lady almoner), lady in centre not identified, Miss W Jackson (registrar).*

landscape with nothing outstanding. A deficit would be countered by a payment from Hospitals Trust and a cumulating overdraft would be met in its own good time by the Hospitals Commission. As events, dampness in the basement and dry rot in the roofspace were less than highlights, each no sooner identified than treated. More exciting was the historical landmark made by energetic attack on the endemic trachoma still lurking in poorer parts of the city. This campaign was successfully mounted by Dr Frank Lavery, here seen as the White Knight who ultimately dispatched that ancient dragon.

Staff members came and went, successive years seeing the passing of the senior Louis Werner after fifty years of service, and of the acerbic Frank Crawley, noted for his entertaining teaching. It was the latter's caustic wit that Surgeon Bill Doolin, himself no mean raconteur, recalled at the next AGM after his death: 'I can remember the shout of laughter that went up from us students at his famous sally that drink, religion, the land question and granular ophthalmia (trachoma) were the four curses of this unfortunate country.'

The evolving social scene was marked in 1938 by appointment of the hospital's first medical social worker, then known as the 'lady almoner', a title regrettably superseded in brisker modern use. (In passing it does to recall how earlier in the century, when women medical graduates were rarer than now, talk of a 'lady doctor' would sometimes stimulate spontaneous ennoblement by patients, so that reference to 'Lady Maxwell' was occasionally heard.) The first lady almoner, Miss Dorothy Connor, set a headline which has been admirably sustained by her successors in the department's fifty years of existence.

That this department provided a unique service from the start is apparent from Council's repeated appreciative references in annual reports, and when in 1947 Miss Connor left to take up a senior position elsewhere, one infers an almost palpable sense of loss. By 1950 the lacuna had been filled by the appointment of Miss Anne Walsh, another outstanding choice, who left only on her marriage to Mr Desmond Douglas, then assistant surgeon in ophthalmology. The present holder of the office, Miss Hilda O'Connell, shows a dedication of service underlined again and again by unsolicited acts far beyond the call of duty.

Meanwhile, during this period of the thirties, routine work in the hospital was proceeding apace. As year after year recorded an increase in the numbers treated, the accurate projection of bed requirements, made so long before, proved fully justified. Clinically, introduction of the slit-lamp was identified with the name of Louis Werner Junior, successful corneal grafting with J B McArevey, neuro-ophthalmology with Alan Mooney, and as mentioned, the extermination of trachoma with F S Lavery. As to the hospital fabric, structural attention included complete interior painting, extra bedrooms for nurses, improved accommodation for domestic staff and provision in all wards of running hot and cold water, surprisingly omitted in the original plan.

In 1939 a major alteration to the front entrance from the street resulted in the 'in/out' arrangement of today. Seemingly the previous entrance had consisted of a single narrow gateway designed for horse-drawn carriages, and accommodating both incoming and outgoing wheeled traffic as well as pedestrians. There was virtually no parking space and the carriageway of rough gravel and sand was considered a hazard to eye patients. Replacement of this with the modern carriage drive was provided by the Department of Local Government. Ironically, one of the few acknowledgements which Council felt impelled to make to this authority, nominally responsible for Public Health matters also, was in respect of this environmental improvement.

The outbreak of World War II in 1939 was reflected in rising prices and shortages, and a necessity to provide against air attack such as threatened even a neutral country. Much time and thought were devoted to ARP (air raid precautions) including provision of a shelter in the basement, protection against incendiary bombs, and modernisation of fire fighting equipment. An extra to the housekeeping budget was an order to purchase up to 100 tons of coal. This was a farsighted provision, since at war's end fuel scarcity reduced some householders to burning their less-regarded items of furniture. In later years Miss Maxwell would reminisce with gratitude on how the Council had saved them all from being frozen to death. The general picture of those years is that while normal functions continued, development was not an option. There was even a happy economy in words when the printed AGM reports omitted the speeches.

With the war drawing to a close came signs of renewed activity. Miss Crowley's sortie to the Irish Red Cross Hospital in Normandy evokes comparison with the earlier war when the British Red Cross had been the magnet. The foundation of an Orthoptic Department broke new ground, Ms Heather Siberry being the first orthoptist.

The year 1947 was the fiftieth anniversary of the Act of Amalgamation. The date was honoured with some ceremony. The choice to celebrate the golden jubilee of the institution rather than of the building, seven years younger, was significant. After all, the Royal Victoria Eye and Ear Hospital had spent the first years of its existence under the roofs of its predecessors, and jubilee demanded acknowledgement not only of its debt to their ideals, but years of its physical existence as well.

19

ACADEMIC ACHIEVEMENTS

Give or take a few years, the golden jubilee of RVEEH, the end of World War II, and commencement of the second half of the twentieth century, were almost coincident. With change to be found in so many dimensions it seems right to see these post-war years as initiating yet another phase in the hospital's story, as indeed they did. By 1950, with human endeavour once again untrammelled, the increase of scientific knowledge, that paradoxical by-product of war, was waiting to be exploited. Humankind was in fact poised for the great leap forward which, still continuing, has nowhere shown advances more dramatic than in the realm of medicine and surgery.

The nineteenth century had seen the special sense disciplines claw their way from empiricism to a dawning practice of method, which the early twentieth century had sought to refine. Only by the thirties was the electric ophthalmoscope replacing a model based on the use of candles as a light source, and only by the forties was it being perceived that the canon of covering both eyes for up to a week after squint surgery in children was needless and dispensable. To cope with the melting of these ice floes of ignorance, RVEEH had assets of material structure, surgical expertise and moral confidence enabling it to face the unfolding era untroubled.

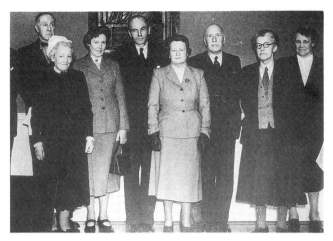

19.1 *Members of Council and staff c.1950. Left to right: Lord Glenavy, president, Miss Allen, matron, Mrs Quin, Mr P J Kelly, Mrs Gordon, Mr Walkey, hon. treasurer, Miss Euphan Maxwell, senior surgeon, Miss Jackson, registrar.*

Since mid-century indicates almost exactly the halfway mark in the history of the new institution, it offers probably the ideal vantage point to look before and after in engrossing the scientific record of RVEEH and its predecessors. For such good reason, an intermission from sequential narrative offers opportunity for an entr'acte of achievements. It also provides better balance between the material story of the fabric, and the philosophical ideals of its foundation, ensuring too that the teaching tradition integral to Dublin medicine is not neglected.

The first intimation of a teaching role in any of the parent hospitals can be found in a certificate issued by Commander Ryall on 28 June 1820, and addressed from the National, then located at No 5 North Cumberland Street. He testified that 'Dr William Kelly, a surgeon in His Majesty's Navy, has attended the practice of this institution for the space of three months, during which time his opportunities of healing disease of the eye have been very considerable. I further certify that he has assisted me in the performance of numerous operations for cataract, closed pupil and various other affections of the eye.' This is the earliest ophthalmic certificate known to have been issued in Ireland, and is fair indication that from the start the primal founder had in mind a teaching institution.

Not until 1845 did the first report from the newly established St Mark's provide further evidence as to teaching. Amidst many aspects of corporate existence requiring mention in this launching document, Wilde took care to announce: 'the attending Surgeon delivers a course of Clinical

Instruction during the winter session in two most important yet neglected branches of medical science.'

At this time also, Wilde was accumulating material for his book on aural surgery. Published in 1853, under the title *Practical Observations on Aural Surgery and the Nature and Treatment of Diseases of the Ear,* it survived initial shafts from some critics, and through its innate good sense and sound principles went on to become the standard text. As mentioned, Wilde's early adoption of the ENT specialty enabled him to become its prophet, the gift of lucid exposition adding to his reputation as a sought-for teacher. In addition to being used in Ireland and England the book was introduced to the United States by one of his American pupils and to Germany and Austria in translation, remaining the accepted authority for generations. The manuscript, in Wilde's own hand, was for many years kept in the hospital library, until its historical value and an overriding need for security led to its becoming housed on permanent loan in the Library of RCSI.

In Wilde's time, reference to St Mark's as a centre for clinical instruction was to recur constantly in successive reports, in what for long was a vain attempt to foster closer relations with the academic bodies. Since academic disdain is notorious, although the hospital Governors repeatedly stressed that a course in ophthalmic surgery was a requirement of the Army and Navy Medical Boards, it was over twenty-five years before it became possible to claim more than that the St Mark's course was recommended by the Board of Trinity College. It was 1871 when at last it could be announced that not alone was St Mark's officially listed in the prospectus of the School of Physic, but that one of its surgeons had been appointed examiner in ophthalmology to Dublin University. At this recognition the Governors' rejoicing was unconcealed.

The distinction of becoming the first University teacher was awarded to Henry Wilson, whose tenure alas would be all too brief. However, his advancement had broken a mould of behaviour and henceforth St Mark's was seen to have joined the Establishment. This connection has never since been broken; even after amalgamation it continued unchecked. Also associated with Wilson's name is the first formal connection of the hospital with RCSI, in whose annals he appears as professor of ophthalmic and aural surgery from 1871, the same year he took office in Trinity. His published work, *Lectures on Theory and Practice of the Ophthalmoscope,* is one of the earliest treatises on this subject. Coming to manhood just at the time the instrument was invented, he had obviously been encouraged to master it by his father, himself never fully proficient in its use. However,

RVEEH has been left happy proprietor of the claim that two of its anointed, Wilde and Wilson, father and son, between them hold authorship of two seminal works in the hospital's specialties.

For the forty years from the mid-seventies until his death in 1913, Swanzy was at the same time both spearhead and focus of academic achievement in Irish ophthalmology; indeed there is a persistent impression that whether regarded in context of these islands or of continental Europe, he remained a giant by any standard. The enduring worth of his textbook has been mentioned. The extent and variety of his dealings with leaders in his field takes physical shape in a unique collection of autographed portraits presented by distinguished contemporaries. Their names in great part spell out the pantheon of ophthalmological 'greats' of the nineteenth century. These photographs, donated by Swanzy's daughters and now displayed in the hospital library, are a reminder to present staff that they come of no mean tradition. Swanzy's nomination in 1888 as Bowman Lecturer was a prestigious choice reserved for those foreseen as achievers of the future.

We know how amply he fulfilled this early promise. An indication by the way had occurred in 1887 with the BMA visit to Dublin when the visiting group of British ophthalmologists had been so deeply impressed by arrangements in the National, then newly moved to Molesworth Street. These men would have been the solemn leaders of the ophthalmic establishment and this visit certainly helped to determine Swanzy's later choice as president of the OSUK, the highest accolade of his peers.

From outside his specialty, the honour of presidency of the Royal College of Surgeons in Ireland, at that time unique for an ophthalmologist, came in 1908, probably influencing the award of a knighthood in the same year. The ultimate tribute came with nomination as president-elect of the ophthalmic section of the International Congress of Medicine in 1913. Death robbed him of this supreme honour, but already he was immortal, by his lifework an ornament to his hospital, his profession and his native land.

In the vicinity of a star of such magnitude, it was difficult during Swanzy's lifetime for his immediate colleagues to shine with full lustre. Yet merit was not to be denied. Where Swanzy was of the nineteenth century, these were men of the twentieth, and they too played a seminal part in the evolution of their specialty. There was Arthur Benson who as describer of asteroid hyalitis, an intraocular lesion of distinctive appearance, was to gain eponymous fame through what came to be called Benson's Disease.

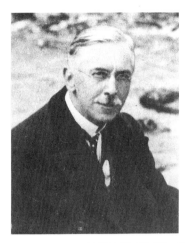

19.2 *H C Mooney, surgeon (1897-1948). The first member of a family that has been continuously represented on the staff of the Eye and Ear Hospital from 1897 to the present day.*

He is permanently honoured in a magnificent bronze and marble plaque in the boardroom of the hospital.

Louis Werner left his mark on the century not only in his editorial and artistic contribution to Swanzy's textbook, which inevitably became 'Swanzy and Werner', but also in giving to Irish ophthalmology such a worthy successor as his son, the much loved L E Werner, so recently lamented, so much missed. Herbert Mooney too, the courteous and the genial, contributed both a son and a grandson to the hospital. All three have added immeasurably to the repute of their Alma Mater. Another protracted record of service dating to the early century embraces not only three generations of the Curtin family, but also the three consultant disciplines they have ornamented, namely, ENT, anaesthetics and ophthalmology – as well as 'Mac' Curtin's distinguished presidency of Council from 1977 to 1979.

Two others making a lasting contribution to Irish ophthalmology were Robert Montgomery and John B Story. The former was a worthy but retiring man who faithfully served hospital and patients without leaving his contemporaries with any impression more vivid than that he was in the habit of wearing a bowler hat. However, in the words of L B Somerville-Large: 'No matter what hat Dr Montgomery wore, when his will was read his contemporaries removed theirs with some respect when they heard he had left £5000 to found an annual lecture in ophthalmology.' This was a very large sum for the period and the Montgomery Lecture, structured to

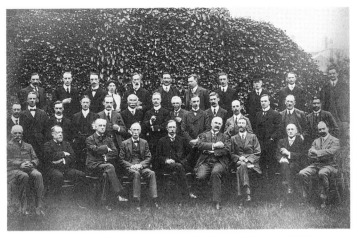

19.3 *Group of OSUK members meeting at the Eye and Ear in 1912, probably the first academic ophthalmic meeting in Ireland. In the back row is Dr Montgomery, wearing a bowler hat.*

alternate between TCD and RCSI, then the ranking medical schools in Dublin, was destined to become in the course of time, the fulcrum capable of advancing Irish ophthalmology to a recognised position on the world stage.

Although leaving no record of personal ophthalmic achievement, Robert John Montgomery was well esteemed by his colleagues, and for a number of years was secretary to the Court of Examiners at RCSI, being himself examiner both in ophthalmology and in chemistry. Nonetheless, he remains overall an enigma, not least for lack of the personal details sought so incessantly by upcoming Montgomery Lecturers. He was a bachelor, living with two sisters who survived him. A personal memoir made by Miss Euphan Maxwell in 1951, some forty years after his death, suggests that the lecture was named in memory of these. However, research for the present record revealed that his father and namesake had in 1853 married a Mary Louisa Prentice. Since it is unlikely that Miss Maxwell knew this was the name of his mother, it is here advanced that, whatever the names of his sisters, the full title of the endowment as established, namely, the Mary Louisa Prentice Montgomery Lecture, was intended to commemorate not the telescoped names of his two sisters, but the mother of all three. That good lady, when she wed her GP husband in 1853, can hardly have imagined how filial devotion would secure the annual exaltation of her name in future centuries.

In 1912 Montgomery attended a convention of the OSUK, doyen of

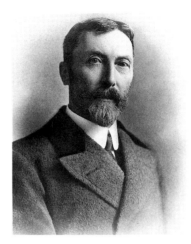

19.4 *John B Story was originally surgeon to St Mark's Hospital. He
became joint senior surgeon on the foundation of RVEEH, where on Sir
Henry Swanzy's death he succeeded him. Sometime president of both
RCSI and OSUK, he was founder of the Irish Ophthalmological Society.*

ophthalmic societies in these islands, which that year had met in Dublin.
(The meeting was held at RVEEH and a surviving photograph shows
Montgomery present, being indeed the only one among thirty-four
participants who is wearing a hat.) This meeting, which had occurred
shortly before his death, may well have inspired the idea that an endowed
lecture might do for Irish ophthalmology what the Bowman Lecture had
done in Britain. While ahead of his time he was brilliantly and
unexpectedly right, though it was to take several decades and the
organisational flair of another individual to catalyse his vision into the
successful entity of today.

In explaining how this came about, it is necessary to note the almost
simultaneous foundation of the Irish Ophthalmological Society, born also
in RVEEH but owning quite another sponsor. The name of Dr John Story
has often been mentioned, starting with his succession to Rainsford at St
Mark's. A respected figure, ranking as joint senior after amalgamation, his
lesser prominence was occasioned only by contrast with the blazing
energy of Swanzy. When on the latter's death Story became sole senior
surgeon, his latent organisational talent came alive, resulting in 1917 in the
formation of the Irish Ophthalmological Society of which he was the
begetter.

It is difficult to do justice to Story, with his work lying for years within
Swanzy's long shadow, but his curriculum vitae shows he was a

considerable person in his own right. The son of a clergyman, educated at Winchester and TCD, he had studied ophthalmology at Zurich and Vienna under Horner, von Arlt and Jaeger, names significant to this day. Back in Ireland he became attached not only to St Mark's but to Mercer's and Dr Steevens' Hospitals, being lecturer in the Ledwich School of Medicine and co-editor of the *Ophthalmic Review*. Family roots in Ulster were responsible for his honorary appointment as High Sheriff of Tyrone in 1911, but his medical stature was growing simultaneously and he was made president of the Irish Medical Association for the term 1913-14.

Having been Swanzy's junior by perhaps a decade, after the latter's death Story was showered with honours. In a society wherein Britain and Ireland were still a single political entity, his peers saw fit to elect him president of the Ophthalmological Society of the United Kingdom for the years 1918-20, an elevation attained by only three other Irishmen ever, one of them Swanzy. Almost certainly, his prospective occupancy of this honorary office underlined for Story the lack of an equivalent society in Ireland, and prompted him to make good the deficiency. For full measure he also acceded to presidency of RCSI, an honour so rare for an ophthalmologist that he and Sir Henry were unique in the distinction.

Thus, by the end of World War I two structures requisite to an ophthalmic establishment had come into being, a society and an endowed lecture. However, while they came from under the same roof, their parentage differed and no formal relationship existed between them. Since the Montgomery Lecture was hedged with legal safeguards, it took a generation before the problem of stitching together lecture and society was to be grappled with and their separate proceedings made to coincide. Appropriately the idea of this union was also born in RVEEH, through the efforts of a talented individual.

This was L B Somerville-Large, universally known as 'Becher', who became secretary of the IOS some time after accession to RVEEH staff in 1934. Irked that society meetings and the Montgomery Lecture were out of phase, with tact and skill he persuaded the Boards of both TCD and RCSI that the society was the proper body to entrust with nomination of potential Montgomery Lecturers. Given the jealous care with which academic bodies cherish their rights, the act of convincing such bodies that on ophthalmic topics, a non-teaching organisation had keener insight than their own, was quite a feat. Time has amply proved this to have been the wisest of decisions, with the teaching bodies retaining their dignity as sponsors, but the clinical practitioners having the acknowledged role of recommending the choice of speaker. By this means it is now possible to

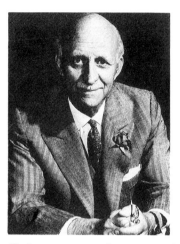

19.5 *L B Somerville-Large, surgeon, historian and prime mover in giving Irish ophthalmology an international dimension.*

pleat the lecture's occurrence into the structure of a meeting, so enhancing the value of both.

First fruit of this innovation came in 1938 when in TCD Professor Lindner of Vienna delivered the first Montgomery Lecture to originate outside these islands. Apart from the intermission caused by World War II, the practice of drawing speakers from far and wide has since prevailed, to the immeasurable advantage of Irish ophthalmology. Somerville-Large's period as secretary was a sort of golden age for the society, witnessing a large increase in membership and a moving forward so that a distinct Irish identity in ophthalmology was recognisable. An all-Ireland body from the start, with membership derived impartially from both parts of the island, in later decades the society adopted the practice of having joint meetings with the national societies of other countries, thus securing for Irish ophthalmology an honoured place in the forum of nations.

Throughout its existence the society was made welcome to use the hospital as a venue for its council meetings. This too was the case with the Irish Faculty of Ophthalmology, a parallel body established in 1957 with the objective of safeguarding standards and conditions of practice, several members of RVEEH staff being also among its founders. In 1992 the changing needs of the turning century determined a merger of these two bodies into a College of Ophthalmologists, subsequently incorporated. Such academic evolution for a specialty now boasting experts countrywide is a welcome development; the role of RVEEH in nurturing the college's constituent bodies is a matter of history.

Members of hospital staff have also been prominent in the proceedings of the Section of Ophthalmology in the Royal Academy of Medicine in Ireland, which encourages participation by junior doctors in clinical presentations. At one time formation of such a section was seen as possibly rivalling IOS interests, but by 1974, with the latter's authority consolidated, the foundation of a section was instigated in a proposition to which the Academy Council in due course agreed. It has proved highly successful as a forum enabling all ages to mix freely.

Somerville-Large's golden age as secretary of the IOS was succeeded in due course by presidency of the society. Later on, in 1962, he became president of OSUK. This was a rare honour for an Irishman in the late twentieth century, when the country had moved to the status of a Republic; it was one achieved by only one other citizen of the Republic, the younger Louis Werner being accorded it in 1974. Both fully deserving of the tribute in the light of their work for Irish ophthalmology, they fittingly joined Swanzy and Story to form the quartet of RVEEH surgeons thus acknowledged by the sister island.

As a mark of a lifelong enthusiasm for his discipline, soon after the war Becher endowed an unusual and useful facility tied to the hospital, the senior surgeons being its trustees. Entitled the Somerville-Large Award, this bounty is reserved for younger consultants at RVEEH to encourage travel abroad, with a view to expansion of clinical horizons. It has proved most valuable in establishing personal links with continental associates. In 1954 for instance, soon after its foundation, it made possible a tour abroad by the present writer, reciprocated in due course by the visit of a young German colleague destined to be a key figure in the evolution of retinal surgery.

The visitor was Dr Gerd Meyer-Schwickerath, who at an IOS meeting held in RVEEH told a fascinated audience of the theory and application of his new approach to retinal detachment. The invention of the therapy known as light coagulation subsequently earned him world-wide celebrity as innovator of a line of thought culminating in the laser. However, he was still a newcomer in 1955, and the paper delivered in Dublin was his first exposition on the subject outside of Germany. Professor Emeritus at Essen until his lamented death in 1992, he cordially acknowledged the Irish visit as the overture to his international celebrity. The occasion stimulated RVEEH to acquire one of his machines, thereby giving new impetus to management of the disease, notably at the hands of Dr Phil Guinan.

At local level in the hospital, Somerville-Large is honoured by an ornamental brass plate erected in the Library during his lifetime. This came as his colleagues' tribute to his efforts in ordering and collating the Library contents, and as donor of one of the fine bookcases housing them.

As a world discipline ophthalmology has a fellowship that ignores frontiers. This, and the fact that so many of the basic nineteenth-century developments in the subject originated in Europe, made inevitable the coming into being of a European Ophthalmological Society, with all the adhering countries represented on its Council. In 1967, Louis Werner Junior, having been for some years the Irish representative, became president of this society, with enhanced prestige not only for himself and his hospital but also for his country. Both he and Somerville-Large were conferred with honorary fellowships of the RCSI in 1965.

It was earlier related how Henry Wilson became the first examiner in ophthalmology at TCD early in the 1870s. Since then the academic position there has always been held by a member of RVEEH staff. With rare intermissions the same is true of RCSI. When in 1985 that college decided to establish a Chair of Ophthalmology, the hospital's nominee, Mr Louis Collum, was appointed. As a result a professorial unit now functions in the hospital, employing a senior lecturer and secretarial staff, with sophisticated teaching amenities. Refresher courses both for ophthalmic practitioners and for GPs are held regularly.

Association with University College Dublin has not been so intimate, owing to long-standing close links between the college and two of the major teaching hospitals, both with active eye departments. An exception to this general rule occurred between 1945 and 1970, when teaching at UCD was under the care of Professor F J Lavery whose major clinical commitment was to RVEEH. With such abundance of clinical material, the college's examinations were based at the hospital during this period. Professor Lavery has been mentioned earlier as energetic in pursuing the final climination of trachoma, persistent till the forties.

A major accrual of prestige occurred in 1966 with elevation of the hospital Pathology Department to national status, as the National Ophthalmic Pathology Laboratory and Registry of Ireland. Resulting from the 1964 appointment of Dr Joan Mullaney as full-time pathologist to the hospital, this reflected her energy and enthusiasm as director, in building what was effectively a new department. Coming from an already distinguished career in general pathology, she established a first-class facility which from the quality of her work quickly rose to international renown. Her selection as specialised moderator for the WHO International Histological Classification of Tumours made her the only Irish practitioner to be so honoured in a list embracing the multiple branches of pathology.

The laboratory acts not only as a service facility for the hospital but also as the reference centre for eye pathology from all parts of the Republic. In the twenty-five years prior to her retirement in 1987, Dr Mullaney produced a constant succession of original papers, bringing lustre to the place as well as to the person of origin. She was a dedicated participant as guest lecturer at international meetings, and her presidency of the exclusive European Ophthalmic Pathology Society in 1987 culminated a period of great academic distinction for the hospital.

Amongst the more recent institutions in RVEEH is the Research Foundation. The brain-child of Dr Alan Mooney, its genesis is described in a later chapter. Since 1975 it has been recognised as a charitable foundation by both the Minister for Health and the Revenue Commissioners, thus securing tax exemption. The vital funding at the start was obtained through annual covenants from the medical staff. Permanent capitalisation was attained by generous support from the two major banks, Bank of Ireland and Allied Irish; the Lions Club of Ireland; the Diabetic Association of Ireland; and personal contributions from the general public. Its multiple range of activities is chronicled in independent annual reports; specially worthy of mention is work on diabetic retinopathy and the causation of retinitis pigmentosa. In the ENT field a feature is the support of laser technology in the treatment of benign and cancerous throat conditions.

20

A NEW AUTONOMY

In evaluating the factors linking affections of the eye with those of nose, throat and ear, common sense suggests they have little in common, and recognition of this will save much fruitless speculation. Viewed objectively, apart from their common siting in the head there is virtually no linkage between these disparate sense organs or common ground in management of their illnesses. True, the normal estuary of lachrymal drainage is via the nose; true again, the headache of sinusitis may mistakenly be assigned to an ocular cause. The grouping together of the disciplines is indeed rooted in tradition, but by and large there is no natural affinity between their functions, and the special sense practitioners hold each to their own terms of reference, meeting as friendly neighbours from adjoining apartments rather than as members of an extended family in a single household.

Historically this was not always so. While Wilde's foundation gave primacy to the eye by twice mentioning it in the title 'St Mark's Ophthalmic Hospital for Diseases of the Eye and Ear', his textbook on aural surgery added to that specialty the weight of a charter document. His practice in the two specialties chimed with the custom of the day, and while he is remembered for eighteen papers on ophthalmological topics, it was by the authority of his famous textbook on ear surgery that he sealed the marriage of the disciplines. His ENT activity is also recalled in the eponymous namings he earned with Wilde's Forceps and Wilde's Incision (used in mastoid surgery and still classical).

His next but one successor, Richard Rainsford, made considerable show of his aural connections, the most resounding of which was designation as 'late assistant in Professor Politzer's Aural Clinique at Vienna'.

It is unquestionable that Swanzy's main dedication was to ophthalmology, and following his war service and later association with von Graefe it is probable he was an early example of the mono-specialist. On the other hand there is no doubt that his contemporary Arthur Benson accepted the dual mandate, since among his appointments is cited that of being surgeon to the Dublin Throat and Ear Hospital, and also of being both ophthalmic and aural examiner to RCSI. Of the twelve clinical papers to his credit, two dealt with ENT topics.

Until the twentieth century however there is little evidence of the practice of ENT work as a separate entity, and in the annals of the combining hospitals the figures for ENT cases form a minuscule proportion of the annual surgical turnover. In the last years of its independent existence, St Mark's, true to the Wilde tradition of statistical analysis, published a series of appendices showing, *inter alia*, the relative in-patient and out-patient figures for cases handled in the respective disciplines during the fifty years since its foundation. Over the whole period, only once did the ENT admissions reach ten per cent of those for eye diseases, the proportion in most years being of the order of five per cent or less. As a contrast, out-patient attendances showed a ratio of only three or four to one in favour of eye cases. A fundamental cause for the disparity between disciplines was lack of lighting techniques which made the fastnesses of ear, nose and throat a *terra incognita* largely inaccessible to surgery. *Per contra,* possession of these techniques is one of several indispensable factors enabling the spectacular work performed in these regions today.

From the foregoing it is easy to see how mono-specialisation in ENT was neither economically nor otherwise feasible at the time the hospital opened. Paradoxically, the individual coming earliest in approach to being an ENT specialist appears to have been one owing major loyalty to general medicine. This was Dr Richard Hayes, a staff physician to Dr Steevens' Hospital who started his association with the National long before amalgamation, being listed as physician for diseases of the throat from 1881 onwards; he continued in this role with RVEEH until his retirement in 1912. Becoming then consulting physician to the hospital, he remained as such until the end of his days. Despite qualifications running to higher degrees both in medicine and surgery, including MD and FRCSI, he

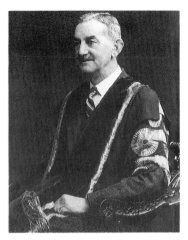

20.1 T O Graham ('Togo'). ENT surgeon 1912-1962. The first Dublin monospecialist in ENT surgery. Initiator with L J Curtin of a separate ENT Department at the Eye and Ear, and founder of the Graham Audiology Clinic.

remained resolutely a physician throughout his career, and was always so described in the hospital records. The role he had played was destined to change after his retirement.

In 1908, a young doctor named T O Graham (to become known far and wide as 'Togo') had served the statutory year as house-surgeon in RVEEH. Just before Dr Hayes retired, Graham applied for and got the new appointment of clinical assistant, with specific responsibility for ear, nose and throat cases. At that time a separate ENT Department did not exist although, unstated in the records, embryonic plans to create one may be inferred. At any rate there followed a swift succession of events. Togo's appointment was made in February 1912. In March came Dr Hayes' resignation, followed in April by Togo's asking to be his successor. This request was denied for one month, although Graham was asked to act as locum, and in May he became Dr Hayes' aftercomer in being appointed surgeon to the Throat Dispensary. This point marked a clear break with tradition, in that Hayes, by definition a physician, was succeeded by Graham, a surgeon. In after-time, Togo always claimed to have been the first practitioner who was exclusively an ENT surgeon.

When Graham joined the Royal Army Medical Corps on the outbreak of war, the embryo ENT Department seemed doomed to suspension for the duration, but moves in 1916 and 1917 indicated a lobby for its revival, a Medical Board resolution to that effect being endorsed by the medical members in Council. The resolution advocated ultimate classification of the

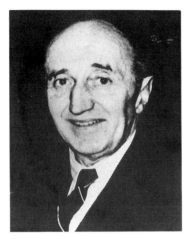

20.2 *L J Curtin, co-worker with T O Graham in initiating a
separate ENT Department. Three generations of the Curtin
family have continuously served on the medical staff from
1919 to the present day.*

staff by specialty, so that henceforth mono-specialisation as ophthalmic
and aural surgeons would be the rule. Since the surgeon to the throat and
ear division held a position above the assistant surgeons, it was urged that
this situation should be recognised in the annual report. If this were
allowed, his name would become formally listed among the surgeons, and
thereby achieve seniority.

This bid for departmental autonomy was successful, and on Graham's
return from the forces he was appointed as senior, thus heralding a new
voice of authority. His co-worker from the start was L J Curtin, some years
his junior but sharing the same dedication to the idea of mono-specialty.
When 'Larry' Curtin also was appointed senior, this provided leadership for
two teams and therefore formation of a separate ENT Department. To
these teams were appointed assistant surgeons in the persons of P D Piel
and P J Roddy, supported by James Hanlon and Margaret Pedlow as
clinical assistants.

Later augmentation in line with vacancies caused by death or retirement
was marked in 1952 by the accession of C D O'Connell, and in 1963 of
Oliver McCullen and Eric Fenelon. George Fennell and William Grant were
appointed in 1967, Andrew Maguire in 1973, while Michael Walsh and
Hugh Burns joined in 1984. The necessity of Jim Hanlon's retirement at an
early age on tragic medical grounds was universally deplored by his
colleagues, in line with an unbounded admiration of the extraordinary
fortitude of his later life.

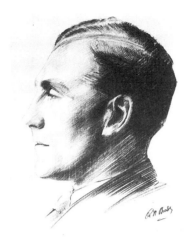

*20.3 C D O'Connell, ENT surgeon from 1952
to 1968. Founding member of the Irish
Otolaryngological Society.*

It only underlines the dichotomy between disciplines that the present writer, an ophthalmologist, is not personally competent to comment on academic achievements of the ENT Division of RVEEH. The material that follows has been furnished by colleagues in that department, to all of whom thanks is extended, especially Andrew Maguire, who wrote the clinical summary.

In the pre-antibiotic era, ENT specialists were primarily concerned with the control of infection, as suppuration deep in the ear and sinuses often led to potentially fatal intracranial complications. The advent of antibiotics, the operating microscope and improvements in anaesthesia allowed the development in the 1950s of reconstructive techniques, most notably in middle ear surgery (tympanoplasty) for otosclerosis and chronic destructive middle ear disease. Later developments led to the restoration of form and function after trauma, and extirpation of malignant disease in the head and neck.

In 1971, George Fennell, who for several years was chief examiner for the FRCSI in otolaryngology, established a joint Head and Neck Tumour Clinic in RVEEH, in conjunction with consultant radiotherapy/oncology colleagues from St Luke's Hospital. This clinic has provided outstanding care to many patients up to the present day and has formed a major advance in management of these distressing conditions, in which careful pre-treatment assessment and long-term follow-up are essential.

The 1970s saw the world-wide expansion of ENT surgery into the neck and facial areas, and even to the skull base and superior mediastinum, a phenomenon reflected in expanded service in the RVEEH Department of Otolaryngology/Head and Neck Surgery. Many of the newer consultants received part of their training in the outstanding department at the University of Toronto, beginning with Andrew Maguire and later continuing with Hugh Burns, Michael Walsh and several subsequent Irish trainees.

The latest techniques of plastic and reconstructive surgery, including external septo-rhinoplasty (nasal reconstruction) and facial and myocutaneous flap were introduced. Operations for patients with laryngeal cancer (to preserve speech in suitable cases), were developed, including supraglottic partial laryngectomy, subtotal laryngectomy and prosthetic tracheo-oesophageal valves.

Hugh Burns, with ophthalmological collaboration, provided an excellent orbital surgical service for patients with exophthalmos (prominent eyes) due to sinus mucoceles and tumours. He also developed special expertise in the surgery of certain tumours of the middle ear, as well as of the salivary gland.

The ENT section of the research unit founded by Alan Mooney investigated the auditory pathways in very young pre-lingual children suspected of being deaf, on a national basis, the technique employed being Brain Stem Evoked Response Audiometry. Michael Walsh introduced relocation of the submandibular salivary ducts in subnormal children with drooling. A cochlear implant programme which he set up unfortunately had to be postponed owing to lack of finance.

Until the late 1980s the ENT Department at RVEEH was the outstanding national department in the specialty, with seven consultants pooling wide expertise and allowing a degree of subspecialisation. It was the tertiary referral centre for the Republic and the main postgraduate centre for the specialty and for the higher examinations of RCSI.

In the late eighties, severe financial cutbacks in the Health Service markedly affected the ENT Department, with halving of the bed complement, failure to replace retiring consultants and loss of ancillary personnel resulting in lowered morale among the highly skilled nursing staff in particular. A most efficient, centralised and economical ENT service was temporarily crippled and this decline had severe political repercussions in subsequent national elections.

Like the Eye Department, over many years the ENT Department at RVEEH has expanded and developed, providing a caring and personal service to countless grateful patients from all over Ireland, who are constantly impressed by the friendly efficiency of this small specialised hospital. A real danger is foreseen that permanent loss of the laboriously assembled structure could result if the services it provides are to be dissipated through 'rationalisation' in the name of progress.

In the teaching area the department is integrated with the higher surgical training scheme in conjunction with RCSI and associated bodies in Britain. When the RCSI established a Professorial Chair in ENT Surgery, appropriately named the William Wilde Professorship, the appointment was awarded to a member of RVEEH staff, Mr Michael Walsh. The RVEEH Department of ENT was the first ENT unit in the country to be accredited for senior registrar training, and is the only one to date which is fully recognised for complete ENT surgical training. Among other records is included that of having introduced the first operating microscope to Dublin.

As founding father of the department, 'Togo' is appropriately commemorated in the naming of the Graham Audiology Clinic. Of immense use to the community, this is a facility for which he early saw the need, pressing for it relentlessly in spite of Department of Health resistance. Its importance was early foreseen as being so valuable for the specialty that enthusiasm for it was translated to a prominent building firm which volunteered to build it at cost, and delivered on this promise. Consisting fundamentally of a sound-proof room wherein hearing deficiency can be calibrated, this purpose-built clinic capably supervised by Ms Judy Nugent now offers a unique resource gladly availed of by other ENT units in Dublin City and beyond.

It was also the ENT Department which largely through the agency of J McA Curtin, strove so long and tirelessly for installation of an X-ray service within the hospital, to replace the previous ad hoc arrangement with private radiologists. When funding was at last made available for this much-needed service, credit redounded not only to the ENT staff which had demanded it and Council which had pursued it, but also to the radiological advice of Dr Max Ryan who fathered the specialised planning. An expensive necessity, its arrival ended years of importuning.

Distinctions enjoyed by members of the department – and in extension by the hospital itself – include the presidency of RCSI on two occasions. T O Graham held the office from 1942 to 1943 and 'Mac' Curtin from 1974 to 1975, meaning therefore that these two, together with Swanzy and Story, have brought the highest surgical recognition to the hospital four times this century. On the international scene 'Mac' Curtin has also been a governor of the American College of Surgeons, Council member for otology of the

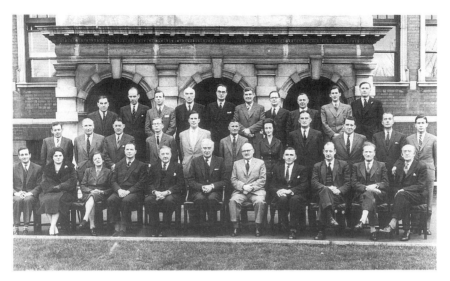

20.4 *Inaugural meeting of the Irish Otolaryngological Society held at the Eye and Ear Hospital, Dublin, in November 1960. Front row: Alec Blayney, Noreen Simpson, Margaret Pedlow, John McA Curtin, F McLoughlin, T G Wilson, David Craig, Con O'Connell, Robert McCrea, R R Woods, Albert P Fagan. Second row: Gus Mulligan, H A Aitken, W Matthews, Colman Fitzgerald, Walter Doyle-Kelly, M J Roberts, Michael O'Brien, an unidentified house-surgeon, C C Corbett, J C Delap, R McNeill. Back row: Eric Fenelon, Rodney England, Gordon Smith, D V McCaughan, Maurice O'Connor, E W R Hackett, Oliver McCullen, H S A Henry, H W H Shepperd, R N Harvey.*

Royal Society of Medicine, and member of Collegium, a scientific grouping drawn from all over the world.

When the Irish Otolaryngological Society was founded in 1960, the RVEEH Department of ENT was at the heart of affairs. Projected as the all-Ireland body which it remains to this day, its germinating committee decided on having a joint secretariat, with representatives from both parts of the island. Representing the southern interest, the late and much-loved Con O'Connell infused his personal chemistry into negotiations, not alone building a vibrant society, but also forming a strong mutual friendship with his northern counterpart, hitherto a stranger. His input to the joint venture was enhanced by Scandinavian insights which lent a continental dimension to his experience. His early death was mourned not alone in RVEEH, but far afield.

In concluding this section a whimsical note may be acceptable. Paddy O'Callaghan, ENT porter for the last four decades and still going strong, recalls from his youth the protocol then attending the surgeon's arrival at hospital. On the Great Man's entry a gong would be sounded, the number of strokes varying inversely with seniority. Having donned his white coat, the surgeon would join his contingent paraded in the hall, made up of a house-surgeon, three nurses and a porter. Before visiting the wards they would process to Matron's office where the Great Man would stop to pay his respects and be regaled with coffee laced with brandy. *Eheu! Fugaces annos!*

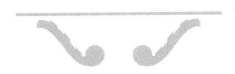

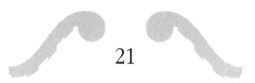

21

THE OLD ORDER CHANGETH...

The Chinese have it that the only certainties in this world are change and death. These pages have often enough witnessed the latter; as for the former, the advance of the twentieth century saw an inevitable alteration in the values and attitudes of society which was to be reflected in hospital affairs also. But the process was gradual, and as the century entered its second half there was no startling upheaval. In time old values would become outmoded and old men would give place to younger, but in 1950 as Lord Glenavy approached his third decade as president of Council it was business as usual. He faced a situation where a combination of rising prices and hospital costs was accentuated by falling subscriptions, while post-war emergence of a Welfare State in Britain threatened to produce a knock-on effect in Ireland.

In public addresses, to his regular theme of an annually increasing deficit he would sometimes add the conviction that Sweepstake funds could not be relied upon indefinitely, reflecting that they were in any case designated for capital use rather than running costs. The Irish medical profession was meanwhile watching with rapt attention the growth of State Medicine across the water, some asserting the scheme would fail, others wistfully reflecting on the security offered to its operators. Here in Ireland the voluntary hospital system was plunging ever deeper into debt, an

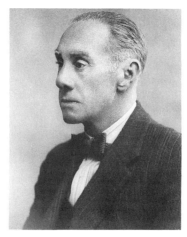

21.1 *Gordon Campbell, Lord Glenavy, president of Council 1931-62.*

ominous sign that continued survival was impossible without assistance. Two of its mainstays, dependence on legacies and on the services of unpaid doctors, were becoming eroded, the one by a shrinking supply of money, the other by envious contrast with our neighbour.

As happens so often the solution lay somewhere in the middle; much painful evolution lay between the post-war scene and now. The date most significant to future change was probably 1947, when with the appointment of Dr Noel Browne as first Minister for Health, there emerged a department no longer shackled to Local Government and in time destined to subsume its creation, the Hospitals Commission. However, because by popular demand the tuberculosis service had prime claim on funding, and since in itself the setting up of a new ministry took time, it was to be years before Council would face the Department of Health as its protagonist of the future.

Meantime, taking the 1951 results as example, Lord Glenavy stated a dire case concisely. From the beginning of 1950 the amount payable towards the deficit had been fixed as the average of the three preceding years. But during 1950 and 1951 costs had risen constantly and every year the prefixed goal was receding. Additionally, although post-war improvements of both drugs and instrumentation were spectacular, they were above all expensive, and without State aid unattainable.

While some hospitals had considerable liquid assets, the modest store of RVEEH was now for the first time exceeded by liabilities. Other institutions being similarly affected, Lord Glenavy warned that without urgent and far-reaching decisions the whole system of hospital financing stood in danger of collapse. In stressing that a country wanting a modern and efficient hospital service must be ready to pay for it, he predicted ward closures unless support were forthcoming. At the same time Sweepstake money was being used to finance the building of provincial hospitals, a practice described as 'filching' by dissatisfied staff in some voluntary hospitals who viewed the Sweep as having been founded to assist their traditional charities, rather than subvent the State in new construction. These old indignations, long since laid to rest, nevertheless merit mention as backdrop to the growth of our Health Service today.

To Lord Glenavy's gloom and doom speech there was no immediate answer, and for some time longer RVEEH continued to limp along financially. Since this is a narrative of its history as an institution and not of its relation to the Health Services, it is needless to follow medico-political vicissitudes in detail down the decades. As Glenavy had implied, the writing was on the wall. In step with the retrospective alms, which year by year came marvellously to retrieve the story of deficit, so too did the State noose tighten and independence become whittled. While the voluntary hospital system survives in name, it exists now at the State's behest and subject to its paymaster's stipend.

It is a relief to turn from the dreary topic of funding to the exciting one of post-war clinical advances. From 1948 on, as a feature of the published report, Council instituted a brief survey of developments, either emergent or in practice, in each of the principal departments of the hospital. Even to those who lived through such changing times, the yearly printed record still gives an animated picture of how much has been achieved in some four decades since the end of World War II. Hence from mid-century on, serving both convenience and logic, the story of RVEEH will be followed on approximately a decadal basis.

One early report on post-war clinical advances sought to emphasise by contrast, setting current results against those of twenty-five years earlier. The beneficial effects of sulphonamides and antibiotics had been amply proved in wartime and were now reflected in a dramatic control of infections. In 1923 there had been fourteen cases of Panophthalmitis, total abscess of the eye, compared with two in 1948, while improved treatment of injuries reduced incidence of the usually blinding Sympathetic Ophthalmia from thirty-nine cases to one. Trachoma, down to some ten per cent of what it had been in 1923, was trembling on the verge of extinction. As for detached retina, for which before 1925 no treatment had

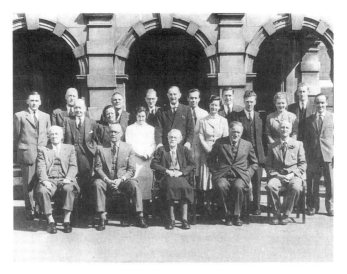

21.2 *Medical staff group, 1957. Sitting: F J Lavery, L E Werner, E M Maxwell, H Tomkin, L B Somerville-Large. Standing: C D O'Connell, P J Roddy, P D Piel, M Pedlow, John Lynham, M O'Connell (house-surgeon), A Hempel (house-surgeon), T O Graham, Roy Naessen (house-surgeon), P M Guinan, T F Roche, T J Macdougald, Sheila Kenny, G P Crookes, D H Douglas.*

existed, sixty-six operations on it were performed in 1948, with a then success rate of some fifty per cent. Corneal grafting was just around the corner, as also was the advent of cortisone, the first of those steroid substances destined to transform the practice of medicine.

In March 1952 the literature carried first reports of surgical insertion of an acrylic lens to replace the patient's cataractous one, and before the year was out three such operations had already been performed in RVEEH. Advances in lachrymal surgery were quickly assimilated, and the new operation of goniotomy for congenital glaucoma found its acknowledged master at the hands of the late Desmond Douglas. In anaesthesia the innovative use of curare was recorded, while towards the end of the fifties, much was made of the purchase of a 'light coagulator', vanguard of a multitude of sophisticated devices making retinal surgery ever more successful. Priced just under £3,000, for some years it ranked as the *dernier cri* in cost and technology. Now superseded by the laser, it survives as a museum exhibit.

In the fifties the ENT Department, elated with .acquisition of an operating microscope, reported several cases operated by the new fenestration technique for relief of deafness, thereby giving entrée to a whole new world of healing. In the same category came the possibility of resumed voice production after laryngectomy for throat cancer. Another ancient enemy of the throat, diphtheria, was being fast eliminated, soon to disappear entirely. The miracle of the hearing-aid was becoming available, but early enthusiasm was tempered by financial obstacles such as huge price differentials between various models and the very high cost of maintenance. Warnings were sounded as to a considerable increase in nerve deafness and problems of industrial and drug-induced deafness. It was also noted that dentures made of the newly introduced acrylic would not show up on X-ray if accidentally swallowed.

For the ENT Department this decade culminated in the opening of the Audiology Clinic, an advance already described. Ranking among what a contemporary description called the 'magical' improvements since the war, it is relevant to record the real fillip given to this project by the unexpected receipt in 1958 of a £500 donation from 'a far-off country', in appreciation of a successful mastoid operation performed years before. In the last year of the decade, despite the use of antibiotics, there were still fifty-one mastoid cases requiring operation, but the character and outlook of the condition had improved materially, with the number of acute and potentially fatal cases declining. Thus as medical history was being made, RVEEH was up with the leaders in rolling back the frontiers of disease.

If the fifties had seen the introduction of so many 'magical' innovations, the sixties were to endure the growing pains of public demand for their provision. All of a sudden good health had in so many cases become attainable that hospital authorities were under steady pressure to deliver it. For perhaps the first half of this decade, the constant problem at RVEEH was a dearth of beds sufficient to accommodate the tide of cataracts and squints seeking admission. Regarded now with hindsight the memory is of departmental frugality in dispensing the funds so badly needed. This economy masqueraded as the laudable prudence of public servants, purse strings being loosened only nearing the end of the decade, when health had become big business for politicians no less than for makers of drugs and appliances.

Lord Glenavy died in 1963, his death ending an unexampled period of thirty-two years as president, by general consent an era of careful budgeting and good husbandry. Entering office when Ireland was classed as a Dominion, he had seen it become a Republic; when he died his stint of office had been served for almost equal periods under each form of regime. Since lords were getting scarcer, one result of his passing was that for the first time since its foundation the hospital's presidency fell to be occupied by someone without any pretence to title.

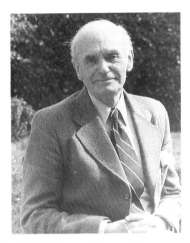

21.3 *Patrick J Kiely, president of Council, 1963-76.*
'A man of unbending Christian principles who worked fearlessly, yet
with humour and kindness, for the greater welfare of the hospital, its
staff and patients.'

Patrick Kiely was a solicitor and shrewd man of affairs who, on becoming president, by the quite irrelevant fact of also being a Catholic, caused an infinitely subtle shift in power balance. While not the first Catholic to occupy the presidential chair, the fact of his being untitled also brought the startling realisation that times indeed were changed. The Crown-centred foundation of the nineteenth century had shifted, to find its axis on People in the twentieth.

Politically this may have been the hospital's finest hour, for despite a changing balance at the top, otherwise all was as before. No one was dispossessed, none overthrown. With great delicacy the new president, who as secretary to Council had been close to Glenavy, steered the same careful course as his predecessor, so engineering a situation of 'Plus ca change, plus c'est la même chose'. Inevitably there were variations of style as between any two captains, but in the conduct of affairs not a shiver revealed the changing of the guard. No doubt the mood of the sixties had something to do with it, when many old certainties were tending to be discarded and with them many old prejudices, but above all, this was a juncture where RVEEH showed a stability bespeaking inner strength at the core.

In this decade the signs of change were livelier than before. A stirring from ancient ways had been seen as early as 1959 when afternoon surgical sessions were sanctioned, at first on a trial basis. As the volume of work multiplied, in both the number and duration of procedures, these extra sessions became an integral function of the hospital, a feature quickly echoed in the annual figures. The total of 2350 ophthalmic operations done in 1960 was exactly double that of 1948 and some three times the number for 1930, without increase in junior staffing.

For some years in the early sixties junior staffing was a friction point with the Department of Health. Repeated requests for permission to appoint registrars were turned down, thus making recruitment of junior house officers more difficult, there being no inbuilt prospect of promotion. The problem was compounded by the fact that for registrars as indeed for nurses and orthoptists too, the salary scale was lower than in the UK, thus further cramping the market. Eventually in 1963 appointment of a single eye registrar was sanctioned, but not before 1964 was a full establishment allowed for both specialties, amounting to ten house officers where initially there had been three.

So insistent was the demand for beds during the sixties that it was decided to convert the men's day room into an extra cataract ward. At foundation, day rooms had been an important facility for ambulant long-stay patients, but being now marginally less vital, altered usage helped to ease a situation where at times bed-occupancy could exceed one hundred per cent of availability.

A further and unusual example of self-help occurred in 1962 when the house at No 61 Adelaide Road, immediately adjacent to the hospital, became vacant. Taking the view that such an opportunity might never recur, T O Graham, by now retired but in the capacity of Council member still a lively presence on the scene, made a personal appeal to staff members, suggesting they might club together and buy it in trust for the hospital. The idea was floated only a few days before sale so that immediate action was necessary. Fired with goodwill, some dozen members of the medical staff put up several hundred pounds apiece, and presto! Council found itself fathering a property it had not even bid for. Initially not overly pleased at being landed in such a situation, it gradually recognised its potential and some time later bought No 62 as well. When No 63 fell vacant a temptation to buy it too was toyed with, but successfully resisted.

The basic idea was a sound one; judicious use of the two houses would free enough space in the main building to put eighteen extra beds on offer. Unfortunately, in this deal the exchequer held the joker, which was permission and funds to make the necessary alterations. With the frugal atmosphere prevailing it was 1968 before these were forthcoming and adaptation could be commenced. Once up and running the premises provided office accommodation, a lecture theatre and flats for resident doctors and senior nursing staff, so justifying the original investment. The subscribers were bought out by the hospital at cost. This plucky venture ended only in the late eighties when a changing admission pattern of shorter bed-stays and quick turnaround made the extra space redundant, and it was decided to sell the houses. Their usefulness ended, they produced a handsome return at auction.

Addressed to an AGM following his accession to office, Patrick Kiely's presidential remarks have continuing relevance today. He had been examining hospital statistics and found that bed cost per annum increased proportionately to the number of beds on offer in an institution. Linking this with the then-recent Fitzgerald Report which advocated larger hospital units and, by corollary, mergers, he compared the process with commercial business takeovers, seeing both procedures as aiming to justify themselves on grounds of rationalisation, efficiency and economy. In his opinion such results rarely followed in business affairs, the effect being rather to diminish human interaction through supplanting personality by a computer cipher. He saw the situation in large hospitals as being analogous, because they tended to minimise the element of personal intimacy existing in smaller ones. This stirring apologia, uttered at a time when the advent of the mega-hospital was still just a cloud on the horizon, showed keen prescience of what effect the Fitzgerald Report would have on future planning.

Meanwhile in RVEEH, as the decade drew to its close, the tempo of work had increased vastly. As already recounted, under Dr Mullaney's direction the Pathology Department had undergone huge expansion into the National Ophthalmic Pathology Laboratory and Registry. Operating theatres had been redesigned, leading to increased efficiency, while a ten-bedded ward had been opened exclusively for squint cases. A second operating microscope had been installed by ENT and the Graham Audiology Clinic was going from strength to strength. The OPD was admitted to be the busiest in Dublin and a well-utilised Glaucoma Clinic had been set up, directed by Dr John Macdougald. Along with these changes the record system was being revised, and the haphazard timing of the past was being replaced by an appointment system.

In other departments, the Nursing School was receiving more applications than it had places. The life-style of nurses was changing, with many choosing to live outside hospital. Innovations included part-time appointments for a speech therapist and a physiotherapist. For the first time a blind telephonist was employed, Marguerite Mitchel who, still happily functioning, has become part of the establishment. Two departments were unstaffed. There was no orthoptist due to lack of a training school in Ireland, and the off-putting salary differential from the UK. With an improved funding policy this problem was to be solved, but not until the next decade. The unfilled vacancy for a medical social worker offered less overt explanation. When established in the thirties under the title of Lady Almoner, this position had rightly been a source of prestige, each monthly report being eagerly scanned by Council. But *autres temps, autres modes,* and vacant for some years in the late sixties, the position had fallen into temporary disfavour, Council demanding medical proof as to the need of it. This situation was definitively resolved in 1972 with the appointment of Hilda O'Connell who revitalised the facility as a model of its kind.

The sixties ended in an aura of hope, with sights set on ever-fresh targets. The difficulty of projecting future needs was perennial; moreover, a realisation that speed of change could nullify improvements was daunting. But RVEEH had never flinched from the difficult, and the new decade came as a challenge.

22

CLINICAL REVOLUTION

The coming of the seventies marked a change of tempo in Council business. Typed minutes replacing the old handwritten ones were symbolic of a new approach for a changing age. As in format, so too in content a fresh urgency was noticeable. Committees abounded, on bed occupancy, on policy, on planning, the latter under the capable chairmanship of Mrs P Maguire whose total contribution to hospital affairs was, and continues to be, outstanding. A memorable accomplishment at her hands was a benefit performance for RVEEH, of Micheál Mac Liammóir's play *Prelude to Kazbek Street,* an event marking the famous actor's acknowledgement of restored sight.

The technical tide was coming in, and flowing with it a passion for change, for novelty, for difference. Piped oxygen was installed in the theatres, and a Recovery Room instituted, both overseen by Alex Tomkin. A welcome and most generous effort by the North Dublin Lions Club was the gift of an installation of pillowphones, enabling each patient to enjoy radio at choice. Accompanying so many improvements were other proposals, some meriting demurral, others occasionally rejection. Efforts to restore the Orthoptic Department were finally brought to success; the aspiration to found an orthoptic school was jointly examined by the hospital and the Department of Health, and agreed by both to be non-viable.

Miss McIntosh retired after a distinguished career as registrar, the position she had occupied being henceforth enlarged to that of secretary/registrar, a subtle alteration signalling the dawning age of professional administrators. The new position was occupied by a rapid procession of incumbents, which halted only on the appointment of Mr David Murphy towards the end of 1969. It would be neglectful to ignore the trojan work of Miss Hazel Church as assistant registrar during those years of transition; not alone that, but also her encyclopaedic knowledge of all things concerning the hospital's administration during long years of service.

Revision of the records system saw much agonising by a retinue of experts in that field. As they conferred, behind them proliferated a space-hungry mountain of paper that for a time threatened to deny house-room to its manipulators, and which ended by gobbling up the now redundant darkroom that had been the heart of Swanzy's Out-Patients. Ultimately, on the suggestion of the late Alex Tomkin, it was agreed to store records that had been unused for more than six years on microfilm. The experience of nearly twenty years has shown the new record system set up by Dr Featherstone and capably supervised by Mairéad Lee to be undeniably efficient; however, those accustomed to old ways will spare a sigh for Swanzy's simple practice of sorting all cases by a colour code, whereby charts in green, blue, yellow and red denoted specific teams of consultants and designated days of attendance. It was probably too uncomplicated for an age anticipating computers, but it worked most smoothly in its day.

In train with the paper explosion within doors, outside there was the obscene proliferation of the motor car, demanding ever more space for parking and restrained only by a hair's breadth from engulfing the blessed half-circle of lawn at the front door, the residue of so much striving by the aptly named Parker. A privately funded tennis court in the grounds offered a staff amenity widely used for some years, until in the end it succumbed to the all-devouring mechanical dragon. In counterbalance, a major advantage resulted from adapting the *porte-cochère* into a reception area, a relatively small modification affording quite disproportionate improvement of access. In line with worsening social mores and the birth of a drug culture, night-time floodlighting of the rear of the building was sadly found to be necessary, although it was successful in repulsing drug thieves with designs on the pharmacy.

The volume of out-patients had always been a particular strength of the hospital, and as the seventies opened it became obvious that the daily routine of those attending by prior arrangement was being compromised by the simultaneous impact of major and minor casualties to which RVEEH by its very name acted as a magnet. Almost overnight the general availability of motor transport had effected an immense increase in the catchment area for acute cases; provision of suitable premises for a twenty-four-hour casualty service was therefore seen as essential. As always, funds were lacking, although for once an encouraging nucleus existed in a grant of £2500 from the Chester Beatty Trust. Though the Department of Health was apathetic, the existence of a partly developed site, taken together with the grant, offered facility to build a separate Casualty Department. Self-help being called for, the balance of funds was raised privately, and a new Casualty erected forthwith, availing of a favourable estimate at a time of rising costs. The ultimate benefit was as expected, despite a frustrating anti-climax at the time of completion. The building having been erected without official permission, there was initially no sanction for staff to run it; perforce it had to stand unused until a new financial year made it possible to employ them. Such are the uses of bureaucracy.

The wisdom and foresight shown in this construction were immediately evident once it was commissioned. Attendance figures during its first year of operation, 1972-73, showed that 32,859 casualty patients were recorded, this being almost half of an out-patient total which over the year had itself increased by almost fifteen per cent. This expanded service for accidents and emergencies was not to be the end of the story: the continuing saga will unfold in its own time.

This period of the early seventies constituted a watershed for all concerned in hospital management, seeing as it did the winding-up of the Hospitals Commission and the virtual disappearance of Hospitals Trust, together with the debut of a major new negotiator. This was Comhairle na nOspidéal, a statutory body drawn from a wide range of interested parties and endowed with ultimate power to decide the staffing establishment of hospitals. It instantly became, as it remains, the ultimate authority in these matters, and in an introductory meeting was recorded as recognising the situation of RVEEH to be unique.

In the nineteenth century local anaesthesia, using cocaine, had allowed operators on sense organs a form of autonomy largely denied to other surgeons. Even so, the role of the anaesthetist had never been ignored; as may be remembered a Dr Beckett, uncle of the playwright, had been appointed in this capacity before World War I. Between the wars Dr Sylvia

Deane Oliver gave RVEEH years of devoted service, the vanguard of a distinguished roll of anaesthetists, many of them women.

As anaesthesia grew ever more sophisticated, so did both eye and ENT surgeons come more and more to rely upon it, a symbiosis culminating in 1971 when a Department of Anaesthesia was established. Dr Kathleen Bayne, working in ENT Theatre, was the first senior anaesthetist in a system employing a cyclic headship of department. With her name must be coupled that of Dr Sheila Kenny, for many years her counterpart in the Eye Theatre and originator of at least one ophthalmic anaesthetic technique to be adopted abroad. In time the department was to expand very considerably to its present establishment of four part-time consultants, together with a registrar working in a recognised training rotation with St Vincent's Hospital. The anaesthetist's function being to produce sleep, and therefore silence, it is regrettably apt that these pages too are silent in allusion to the personal contribution of so many individuals in the hospital's total achievement. This implies no forgetting of their deeds; rather must each name on the list of anaesthetists in this book itself infer remembrance on the roll of honour.

As the discovery of X-rays in 1895 almost coincided with the foundation of RVEEH in 1897, it is hardly surprising to find that there was no initial provision for radiology. In its early years this discipline was regarded with some awe as being not a little dangerous for its practitioners, apart from which many ingenious techniques which make it now so valuable had yet to be developed. As a result there grew up at RVEEH an *ad hoc* arrangement to send cases to private radiologists when the need arose. The usage was at first not impractical, having developed at a time when referrals were infrequent. Since radiologists on the panel all practised near the hospital and patients were almost always ambulant, they were easily conveyed by taxi. Naturally as time moved on the system was found to be ever more clumsy and time-consuming, but since always there were other demands on funding, provision of so expensive a facility awaited the grace and favour of the State.

From 1973 onwards absence of such a department was recognised as intolerable in a modern hospital, a situation aggravated by the foreseeable retirement of most of the private consultants providing the service. From this date forward the matter arose constantly in Council business, but five years were to pass before agreement in principle to provide it was yielded by the Department of Health. More water was to flow under the bridge before the facility eventually materialised in custom-built premises adjoining the OPD, an event to be mentioned in the next chapter. The initiative for construction came from Mr Justice Griffin and 'Mac' Curtin who persuaded Council to act, and aided by the strenuous efforts of Messrs Whitaker, Donnelly and Byrne, it at last succeeded in having agreement in principle translated into action.

So many changes and developments occurred in the seventies that collation of them is complex. A portent of the future was the establishment of a Retinal Unit under the direction of Maurice Fenton, with Geraldine Kelly as research fellow, soon to be a consultant. A wistful link with the past was seen in protracted negotiations with St Ultan's Hospital, which surviving the death of its founders, sought a variation of identity as newer facilities outstripped it. Unfortunately no workable plan could be devised, and Kathleen Lynn's admirable institution was finally closed, its premises now forming the Charlemont Clinic.

Alan Mooney's campaign for establishment of a Research Department was surely the largest single enterprise of this period. It was all the more remarkable in being a work of his so-called retirement years, when he had ceased to be engaged in hospital practice. Commencing in 1975 with the institution of the RVEEH Research Foundation as a charitable body, action started the following year with the relatively modest purchase of a mobile home; installed in the hospital yard, it provided a physical base for what as yet was the personal dream of the founder.

Only on reading the contemporary Council records does the magnitude of Mooney's achievement become apparent. It is then one recognises that his iron will in pursuit of a private vision was not dissimilar to Swanzy's. Within a few years he saw erected the first permanent addition to RVEEH since the Harvey Lewis Wing fifty years before. The purpose-built unit is physically integrated with the main building and through the architectural skill of Brian O'Connell blends happily with it in stylistic conformity. Despite administrative existence as a separate foundation, its services are at the disposal of hospital staff as needed. In addition to a medical director, it is staffed by a research fellow, two technicians and two part-time secretaries. Services offered include electroretinography, dark adaptation testing, the sophisticated Farnsworth-Munsell Hundred Hue test for colour vision, and other advanced tests in extension of standard amenities available in the main hospital.

However, Alan Mooney's achievement was confined neither to this working unit nor to its physical manifestation. Uniquely he also secured the unit's future funding by substantial benefactors, something never before attained in the hospital's history. It was only fitting that the single-minded determination of this most modest of men was acknowledged in dedication of the completed work as the Alan J Mooney Research Unit.

During this decade also, new arrivals on the staff heralded the harvest of the future. In 1969 had occurred the lamented death while still in his prime, of T F Roche, an amiable and popular colleague who had organised modernisation of the Eye Theatres in the sixties and whose particular surgical interest had lain in corneal grafting. Henceforward new ophthalmic appointments would feature a choice of incomers on a special-interest basis, enabling the hospital to be armed at every point, as befitted the largest grouping of ophthalmologists in the Republic.

Already a solid corpus of general ophthalmic practice was available at the hands of existing staff members. T J Macdougald originated the Glaucoma Clinic, which he built into a most useful facility. The present writer inherited care of the Orthoptic Department, which moribund for a time, needed slow nursing back to a now healthy state. John Blake collated facts and figures as to glass injuries in road-traffic accidents, a work of immense importance which after patient years bore fruit in legislation securing elimination of toughened glass windscreens in favour of laminated ones. The forte of Joseph Walsh lay in paediatric ophthalmology, that of Alex Tomkin in contact lenses. In such an era of challenge new methods and the hands to execute them were always in demand, something particularly true for the rapidly advancing management of retinal detachment. This disease, incurable prior to 1925 when it was the ugly duckling of eye surgery, had become the success story of the later century. While eschewing invidious mention, the names of D H Douglas, P M Guinan and F D McAuley had long been noted for interest and expertise in this area. From 1967 a gifted new surgeon in the field appeared in the person of Maurice Fenton.

In January 1971, two new appointments lent added potential to the work force. Having made their mark as house officers, Louis Collum and David Mooney were welcome recruits to the team, and quickly showed the colour of their interests, the former in all aspects of corneal surgery and diagnosis, the latter in the field of fluorescein angiography and fundus photography. In the years ahead both were to flourish mightily. The corneal interests of Louis Collum were to expand into the larger activity of the RCSI Chair of Ophthalmology, of which he became the distinguished first occupant. In the field of angiography, it is quite remarkable how, starting from scratch, David Mooney has synergised the two divisions of photography and angiography into a single indispensable diagnostic tool. The entire space of the former casualty section is now occupied by this department. In David's lexicon and that of Stephen Travers, his photographer and ally, the unobtrusive quest for perfection is endless.

These advances were of course not instantaneous. The remainder of the decade was largely a tale of progression by inches, as more difficult budgeting demanded an annual priority list of instruments for purchase. One example of Council's determining role occurred when an expensive camera for intraocular use was urgently needed and departmental sanction was delayed unduly. To its great credit, Council advanced from its slender private funds the £9000 needed to buy it.

By this time the wheel had almost come full circle, with departmental policy impinging more and more on the hospital's freedom to act independently. The Fitzgerald Report now gradually being implemented had at its heart the regional development of health services. One result of this was that RVEEH, which on foundation had drawn patients from most of the thirty-two counties, now became officially the Regional Eye Centre for the Greater Dublin area south of the Liffey. This paper designation fell far short of its continuing significance through being the largest ophthalmic establishment in the Republic, both in size and staffing, and also the heritor of an ophthalmic tradition of nearly two centuries. Furthermore, as seat of the National Ophthalmic Pathology Laboratory and Registry and of the prestigious Alan J Mooney Research Unit, it remained pre-eminent.

As the eighties dawned, the colossal clinical expansion of the Health Service and its corresponding growth in political importance provoked baleful regard by the planners, of a unit which failed to fit an idealised tidy pattern. The specious argument was advanced that small and specialised hospitals had no place in the system, a plea belied on many counts. But as the creeping Utopia undermined one historic foundation after another, RVEEH was not to be spared its searching attention.

23

THE PERSISTING CHALLENGE

The role of president, which Swanzy and his peers had weighed so finely in the early century, remained no less critical for the hospital in the later decades. When P J Kiely died in office in 1976, he had been a Council member for thirty-one years and president for thirteen; between them he and Glenavy had shared nearly fifty years of office. He was followed by John McAuliffe Curtin who, with a proven record for leadership, ably guided the fortunes of Council until 1979, when he was succeeded by Mr Henry Boylan, also distinguished as an administrator. These two gentlemen each gave two years from already crowded lives in unstinted service to the hospital.

Among many developments during these last years of the seventies, most notable was the setting up of medical liaison with St Vincent's Hospital, lately translated from its parent site at St Stephen's Green to the new building at Elm Park. There, as a first fruit of the Fitzgerald Plan and as the only modern general hospital south of the Liffey, it stood ready to complement what RVEEH had to offer.

Echoing the canon that medical science is a unitary discipline, this liaison of a specialised hospital with a large general one provided a good working arrangement which granted RVEEH access to a full range of skills whenever needed. Evidence of Comhairle na nOspidéal's overall strategy

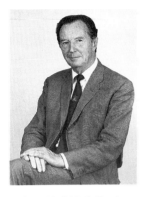
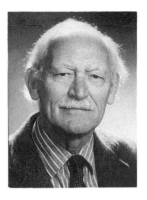
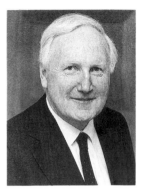

23.1 *Mr J McA Curtin, president of Council, 1977-79.*

23.2 *Mr Henry J Boylan, president of Council, 1979-81.*

23.3 *Mr John Donnelly, president of Council, 1981-87.*

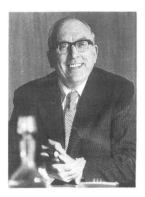
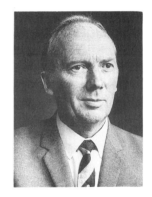

23.4 *Dr T K Whttaker, president of Council, 1987-1991.*

23.5 *Mr Justice Frank Griffin, president of Council, 1991 to date.*

as to staffing was apparent in its structuring of new appointments. Henceforth these would be made only on the basis of economic viability, each new appointee being assured of the means of livelihood through sufficiency of guaranteed sessions. This sensible feature bore the corollary that appointments embracing more than one hospital must not straddle the north/south divide of the River Liffey, a reasonable provision considering the physical difficulty of bi-location across an intervening stream.

The practical result of this for RVEEH was that any new joint appointments would be based south of the river, effectively predicating its alignment with the three southside hospitals, St James's, St Vincent's, and the Adelaide. Exceptional to this rule was the case of the Midland Health Board, which provided for RVEEH a hinterland containing some quarter of a million people. Recognising a relationship by contiguity, Comhairle found it appropriate to offer a joint consultancy between region and special sense hospital, with the incumbent based on the latter. This new pattern, suitable to the needs of a new age, was made individually applicable to both Eye and ENT Departments. Denise Curtin, heralding the third generation of her family to hold consultant status in RVEEH, became the first holder of this position in ophthalmology, while Hugh Burns, ENT consultant from 1984, corresponded for his discipline.

The advent of the eighties witnessed large changes taking place within a short span. At the end of 1979 occurred the sudden and lamented death of Desmond Douglas while still in office, his passing depriving the hospital of a tower of wisdom and experience. Within months came the retirement of Harris Tomkin after an association of fifty-four years with the hospital. Three years later his son Alex was carried off untimely; the gallantry of his last year when, facing the inevitable he lived every moment left to him, will long be remembered.

Within the first half of the eighties occurred the scheduled retirements of T J Macdougald, P M Guinan, G P Crookes and F D McAuley from the Eye side and J M Curtin from ENT. A link with St James's Hospital came in 1981 with Hugh Cassidy taking a joint appointment between it and RVEEH. His commitment to the latter when senior registrar was remembered and lent to his promotion a flavour of homecoming, while the connection with St James's added to RVEEH a usefully enlarged sphere of influence.

Other new arrivals came in the persons of Paul Moriarty in 1983, Peter Barry in 1984 and Martin O'Connor in 1986. Each of them offered special skills, respectively in surgery of the orbit, of the retina and vitreous, and of motility disorders, each likewise being attached to a southside general hospital. To ENT came Hugh Burns and Michael Walsh, augmenting a team depleted by the retirement of Oliver McCullen and Eric Fenelon.

Miss Prunty, who had dignified the position of matron for twenty-five years, likewise reached retiring age, being succeeded by Miss Augusta Fitzsimons, who infused the office with the unique enthusiasm of her own personality. This general post, in a way reminiscent of the abrupt changes at St Mark's almost exactly a century before, left the clinical establishment markedly altered. The upheaval was matched by a similar stirring in Council when, on Mr Boylan's retirement as president in 1981, Mr John Donnelly was elected to succeed him.

The new president, a Council member since 1966, had become its treasurer in the seventies. To a legal qualification he added a career in accountancy which showed financial skills that were outstanding. He brought to the presidency a formidable driving force, aiming to introduce fresh blood in Council's membership, and increasingly involve younger consultants in its operation. Additionally, he pledged a firm resolve to raise those funds whose lack had been the hospital's core problem for almost a century. To this objective he applied himself with an intensity that was awesome. Having set a prime target of almost a million pounds, he relentlessly pursued, and achieved it within some six years, whereupon he relinquished office. The hospital owes him an immense debt for untiring efforts spent selflessly in its service, as well as for their enduring results seen in elements of new building that arose during his presidency.

The activity of the early eighties was phenomenal. By 1982 the X-ray Department was already a-building. Awaited for generations, the need for it had been conceded by the Department of Health in 1978. Construction was completed in 1983, and with the appointment of Dr James Griffin as radiologist, in March 1984 the unit came into operation, swiftly proving itself both as to need and efficacy. During its first full year nearly ten thousand X-ray examinations were carried out, and fresh applications of techniques suitable for special senses were already being identified. The service aspect of ocular ultrasound was taken over from the Research Department, and a notable advantage was found in the facility's physical closeness to Casualty.

While the X-ray development had been funded by the State, it was clear that the hospital's next aspiration held no prospect of State help of any sort. In these circumstances, under the dynamic drive of the president, an intensive fund-raising campaign was started. Managed like a military operation directed at a named target, cash was sought from all possible sources, through organised events, by collection and subscription, but most of all by covenant. It was recognised that only by self-help could the hospital's perceived mission be attained; having a clear-cut prime objective, no time was lost in its pursuit.

This objective derived from the fact that by now the demand for a twenty-four-hour Casualty presence made enlarged accommodation imperative for this service, proving incidentally how necessary had been the *ad hoc* solution of the seventies. The fact that the 1973 building had been crammed almost from the moment of completion was central to the case for its replacement, an argument endorsed in 1983 when the annual report highlighted the unit's tenfold increase in usage since its inception ten years before. In a way this unequivocal message made easier the task of fund-raising, since the existence of so specific a target abolished any need for lengthy justification. Conjoined with this was a further aim to acquire an enhanced range of out-patient equipment, the combined objectives being nominated Phase One of a fund-raising exercise destined to occupy much of the eighties.

If covenants and subscriptions were secured by committee work, action on the ground lay with well-wishers, whose numbers became apparent only as Dubliners came to realise the needs of their beloved 'Eye and Ear'. The spontaneous donation of an ultrasound machine jointly by the Irish Transport and General Workers' Union and the Irish National Bookmakers' Association was gratifying both in its intrinsic usefulness and as a symbol of how the populace cared. The gift showed how accomplishment is primed by enthusiasm among individuals, the trail blazers in this case being the stalwart Jimmy McLoughlin and his friends in the bookmaking fraternity. Their effort lit a torch for many others, stimulating ventures such as sponsored runs, art exhibitions and raffles, among these being one for a beautiful handmade patchwork quilt which raised the striking total of £13,000.

Selective mention in no sense belittles the multitude of unsung helpers, and no one is likely to begrudge special praise for the quite splendid contribution of the Tallaght Fire Brigade. From among its members Jim Cleere and the members of 'B' Watch organised a sponsored drive in a vintage Rolls Royce fire engine over the circuit Dublin-Cork-Limerick-Dublin. Sped on their way by Dublin's Lord Mayor they returned with the sum of £12,700 in their collecting boxes, a significant addition to the fund for costly new instruments. This collection augmented a donation of £25,000 from the Marie Curie Foundation to secure a Yag laser, equipment vital to any modern eye hospital.

When reporting this purchase among a list of other expensive instruments, the president was at pains to indicate that while bought with funds raised privately, these goods were subjected to VAT at twenty-five per cent, so that in effect the taxation code was penalising the hospital in respect of funds donated charitably. The point was well made, that while the voluntary hospital ideal still had fire, the odds were staked against it.

The new Accident and Emergency building was opened in January 1986. At last of a size sufficient for its needs, this too was paid for by funds from the recent initiative. Built in a year described as being 'most difficult' for the hospital, when even running expenses were reduced to meet Government cutbacks, the enterprise demonstrated sturdy confidence in facing the future, as well as an admirable sense of responsibility. Indeed it could be proved that the hospital was operating at an efficiency factor thirty-six per cent greater than any other specialist or general hospital in the country, a claim quite in keeping with the record of tightly reined management throughout RVEEH history. Here was surely solid cause for satisfaction, in a voluntary body proud of its past, conscious of present achievement and eager for the future.

But alas, this was to be a high-water mark for years to come. Sadly the very report which carried the account of so cheerful and forward-looking an occasion, also gave details of State thinking as to the hospital's future. It was signalled that the ultimate price for all the years of financial support was to be loss of identity; in the jargon of our times, there is no such thing as a free lunch. The president described how over the years Comhairle na nOspidéal had published two discussion documents on future development of both Eye and ENT services in Dublin. To each of them RVEEH had made a detailed response backed by statistical and financial evidence, clearly showing its very substantial contribution to its specialties. It had factually shown operation of the Eye and Ear to be more economical and efficient than would be a service located upon the campus of a general hospital, as advanced in the documents. Although by definition these documents implied there would be further discussion, in the event no opportunity for verbal amplification of the Council's written replies had been given.

When the Minister had visited the hospital in November 1985, he had spoken of his department's policy to rationalise the number of units, providing the same or similar services at multiple locations in Dublin; he also spoke of a need to curtail bed numbers within the two specialties. In response Council had indicated its concurrence with such economy, made evident by measures such as introduction of day-care, and ward closure during holiday periods, and had offered reasons why it would be in no one's interest to transfer elsewhere services already comprehensively and economically provided at RVEEH.

Mr Donnelly then described the department's intentions. It proposed a plan which effectively would disperse the services of RVEEH, Eyes to St Vincent's campus, ENT to St James's. As president he voiced Council's concern, deeming the proposals to be costly and impersonal, imposing burdens on both patient and taxpayer. He suggested it was inconsistent with rationalisation to fragment specialist services in a way which would increase their cost. In his opinion not only would patients be less well served but running costs relying on exchequer subsidisation could be doubled or trebled, with capital cost quadrupled. Speaking as a practising accountant his conclusion was that it was clearly not possible to locate the existing combination of specialties at more than one centre in Dublin without duplicating their cost.

It has never been clearly defined how this decision was arrived at. Representing the choice of theory over practice, it accepted the special sense disciplines as distinctive entities, but seemed to insist their most effective practice must lie in co-habitation with the extended medical family under the roof of a general hospital. This idealised hypothesis has greatest weight when the entirety of a hospital is being set up from scratch; it loses power when a given service is pre-existing.

Especially is it debatable in respect of ophthalmic hospitals, the paragon of Moorfields being the outstanding example of autonomous existence, although others, less well known, are no less eminent. Within the last five years Bristol, Dublin's cousin over the centuries, and just four years senior, with an ophthalmic tradition dating to 1810, has reasserted ophthalmic autonomy in the launching of a new eye hospital. When, as with RVEEH, there is additionally a monumental dimension, the case acquires another aspect, deserving evaluation via different parameters, including history. It is easy to accept that almost certainly such factors were not even recognised, let alone considered, before decisions were taken. With these factors now stated, it is reasonable to claim they make a difference.

These 1986 proposals saw the unfolding of a programme which, if implemented, would unravel the thriving achievement of a century, and the tradition of almost two. Coming at the climax of a highly successful fund-raising effort which provided a new Casualty Department through private endeavour; coming also in that decade when the State itself had seen fit to provide a costly X-ray Department in premises it was now proposing to quit, the decision was seen as containing innate contradictions.

Adding to the frustration and dismay shared by staff, patients and public, the fund-raising exercise came to an end. A survey commissioned by Council had disclosed that success for an intended Phase Two, to be directed towards the United States, would have been doubtful. Coincidentally, Mr Donnelly, who had generously added an extra year to the five he had pledged to leadership, completed his term as president.

Succeeding him was Dr T K Whitaker. With repute second to none as a public servant, he lent major strength to RVEEH at this difficult time. Initially as chairman and later as president, leadership of Council brought him into difficult years, through which he guided his charge with wisdom and integrity, while alas not managing to alter the pre-set course he had inherited. His distinguished term in office ended in 1991 when he was succeeded by Mr Justice Griffin, long a Council member, whose judicial record promised maintenance of justice and right.

It is now six years since the proposals for the Eye and Ear's future were announced. Difficulties in the scheme soon became evident when examination on the ground showed the plan to be incapable of immediate execution. Consultation with authorities of St Vincent's Hospital revealed that without new buildings the proposed transfer could not be accommodated. Due to a perennial shortage of funds for other projects, financial provision for such buildings appeared unlikely in the near future. Therefore the proposed change remained indefinitely suspended, a sword of Damocles poised to fall at a date unstated.

More recently, inspection of the hospital by a new minister has led to hope of continued protraction by his department, based on clear absence of the funding necessary for a major house-moving operation. A loophole remains that expediency may yet allow the optimum scenario to prevail and that after so long a travail, this historic building may ultimately retain the use for which it was originally built.

At this point the present writer begs leave to offer a personal view, invested with no more authority than dedication to an institution he has served throughout his working life and which he believes to be entitled to honourable survival. The proposition advances a plea resting on the labours of past generations yet cognisant of the pride of those to come, who well may spurn actions done in this age if they deprive them of an irreplaceable tradition based on an historic site. It recognises and respects the Council's obligation to comply with the ruling authority, a pragmatic attitude dictated by necessity.

But no such restriction invests an alternative argument fired by passion rather than politics. It is at least certain that what follows represents not merely the pipe-dream of one individual, but the wish and aspiration of many more for whom the Eye and Ear Hospital on Adelaide Road is not just another institution but the embodiment of an ideal and a focus of loyalty. The received mandate of this book was to record the hospital's story, but as chapter after chapter unfolded, so did indignation grow lest an achievement entailing so much loving sacrifice should be allowed to vanish unwept or without public airing of a case which has no other forum.

The title of this book was not idly chosen. While the life and work of

Sir Henry Swanzy raised in the Eye and Ear Hospital a spontaneous memorial to his genius, in erection of its physical structure he may hardly have been aware of creating a powerful symbol of much else besides. Inheriting as it does the traditions both of Ryall and of Wilde, with each of whom he identified, his building has inevitably become also a monument to them and their original foundations, from which phoenix-like it arose.

Furthermore, through provenance from Utrecht and the school of Snellen it represents an umbilical attachment to the main corpus of European ophthalmology. Indeed in its own fabric it goes far towards being a spontaneous monument to that important discipline. In its style the building is a national treasure, a unique exemplar of its period, and a shrine of the noble sciences for whose practice it was specifically erected.

Looking then to its future, it may be asked how serious was the intent in Dublin's proclaimed identity as European City of Culture in 1991. If indeed this claim were in earnest, in how far can it now be justified to sever from its ordained use a monumental building having European provenance? It is here argued that needlessly to walk away from a building specifically dedicated as Swanzy's memorial is to slight the memory of a noble humanitarian, a great Irishman and a giant among giants in those stirring years when Europe fathered the growth of ophthalmology into the clear entity it is today.

Disregarded in a projected quitting of the Adelaide Road building is the entire historical tradition this book has sought to bring to notice. Its story of great endeavours in a worthy cause has featured the accumulation, like a coral reef, of an uncountable number of individual acts into a splendid whole. The pennies of the poor, a myriad of tuppences and threepences, whose donors stand acknowledged by name in the printed records, were surely not given for the building to be yielded to other use.

It is not as though without merger the institution would remain unviable. Even with restricted financing it is presently giving a first-class clinical service with an unquantifiable bonus in its smallness. Small indeed is beautiful, and it is unarguable that the quality of tender loving care, the backbone of good nursing, exists in the present institution to an exceptional degree, as endless praise from its patients gives witness. It is apparent that all grades of staff are content in the present location. Together with the cost of relocation in a building as yet unerected, must be counted the vacating of a purpose-built and centrally located edifice still not a century old, albeit now in need of some refurbishment.

The projected quitting of this noble and well-managed institution implies not only the surrender of an asset, but the inevitable corollary of yet more expenditure on new structures that this small nation can ill afford. There will be no shortage of envious eyes to fasten on this lovely building if vacated, nor in such case, of cash to adapt it to other use. The imagination would recoil in consternation if the physical embodiment of all Swanzy's striving were to end, not in the bang of medical advancement, but in the whimper of an office building.

It is hoped these thoughts may challenge the reader, and evoke recognition that planning is for people and not vice versa. In the long run all planning is rooted in theory, and if theory is to override dutiful remembrance of the past it becomes itself an object for criticism. Nor is the theoretician immune to rash judgement; witness the hasty and soon regretted abandonment of the Harcourt Street railway line, which now so reproaches its destroyers and which also, if restored in modified form (as may well happen), would further emphasise the already existing centrality of the Eye and Ear Hospital.

Standing on the threshold of a new European order and of a new century, it is all the more necessary to cleave to our heritage, to fear the monotonous growth of uniformity in a shrinking Europe, and the dwindling of what is unique. If this history has demonstrated that the building that is the Eye and Ear Hospital shows such uniqueness, in concept, in utilisation and in what it stands for, then it will not have been written in vain. We have earned too well of nineteenth-century Dubliners to sanction dereliction of their monuments in the twentieth.

APPENDIX A

The following History of St Mark's Hospital was published in the hospital's fifth report (1851). As a source document for the present work, it has been extensively drawn upon in the text, but in view of the minute detail afforded it is here given in full for the benefit of historians.

HISTORY OF ST MARK'S HOSPITAL

As this Institution is now fairly established, some account of its origin and history will not only prove interesting in itself, but serve to exhibit the claim which it has upon the citizens of Dublin for support. At the early part of the last century, the Medical Charities of Dublin consisted of;–

The Charitable Infirmary;–on the Inns-quay, founded and endowed in 1728, by six surgeons of the city of Dublin–Messrs. George and Frederick Duany, Patrick Kelly, Nathaniel Handson, John Dowdall, and Peter Brenan. It was originally situated in Cook-street, and could accommodate but four intern patients. On being removed to the Inns-quay, the number was increased to forty. Upon the erection of the Four Courts, this institution, which was the first hospital established in Dublin, was removed to Jervis-street, where it still exists.

Steevens's Hospital;–erected by property bequeathed for that purpose by Dr Richard Steevens, an eminent physician in this city, and opened in 1733.

Mercer's Hospital;–erected and endowed by Mrs Mary Mercer, in its present locality at the end of Stephen-street, in 1734.

The Hospital for Incurables;–established by the "Charitable Musical Society of Crow-street," in the year 1744. In 1760 it stood on Lazer's-hill, now the lower end of Townsend-street.

The Hospital for Poor Lying-in Women;–in George's-lane, (now South Great George's-street) erected by Dr Bartholomew Moss, in 1745, and now the Dublin Lying-in Hospital, Rotunda, Sackville-street; the first of the kind opened in the British dominions.

St Patrick's Hospital;–founded by Dr Jonathan Swift, D.S.P., for Lunatics and Idiots, opened in 1757.

The Meath Hospital;–originally opened in Meath-street, 2nd

March, 1753, for the benefit of the Poor Artisans in the Earl of Meath's Liberty.

The Lock Hospital, in George's-lane;–(originally opened in Rainsford-street,) the first of the kind in this kingdom, likewise owed its origin to the bounty and benevolence of a medical man, having been "instituted in 1755, by Surgeon Doyle." A similar institution was founded by subscriptions, and opened in King-street, Oxmantown, in August, 1758.

The Infirmary, in James's-street, for the Sick and Wounded Soldiers of the Army;–which existed in 1757, did not properly belong to the Medical Charities of Dublin at that period, no more than the present Royal Infirmary, in the Phoenix Park.

St Catharine's Hospital;–in Meath-street, for Poor Surgical Patients, opened 17th August, 1758, was afterwards incorporated with the following:

"St Nicholas's Hospital, or the New Charitable Infirmary;–in Francis-street, the first of the kind established in that populous part of the city, was," as we learn from the almanacs of the period, "begun in Cole-alley, Meath-street, 26th October, 1752. But that place being insufficient for the numbers daily resorting thereto, the surgeons took a large and convenient house in Francis-street, capable of receiving forty intern surgical patients. It was opened upon the 1st April, 1753." Regular attendance was given, both in Physic and Surgery, every morning, from 8 until 10, by Drs Patrick Kelly, John Taaffe, and Edward Jennings, physicians; Peter Brenan, Cusick Roney, Thomas Mercer, James Dillon, and Edward Walls, surgeons; who attended alternately without remuneration. Portions of the original building still exist, at Nos. 129 and 130 Francis-street, and in the old dilapidated houses yet remaining in Infirmary-yard behind these premises, and running parallel with Swift's-alley Church. It appears to have been established chiefly through the instrumentality of the physicians and surgeons belonging to it. It was supported by subscriptions, and the interest of a fund raised by lottery. What may have been the amount of the sum acquired by the lottery we have not at present any means of ascertaining, as the original Minute Book of the Hospital has long since been lost sight of, but we·know that it was vested in Navigation Debentures, *the interest alone of which was employed for the purposes of the Hospital. In the year 1759, the Rev. Dr John Smith bequeathed to this charity a Kinnegad Road*

Debenture, No. 290, for £50. This property, together with the residue of the fund raised by the lottery, still appertains to the institution.

In 1787, St Catharine's Hospital already alluded to was united with the Charitable Infirmary, and the name of the latter changed to that of "The United Hospital of St Nicholas and St Catharine." As appears from the almanacs of the day, many of the most celebrated physicians and surgeons of Dublin were attached to this institution during the latter part of the last century, and "all served without fee or reward." Again, we read that "from 1st Nov., 1762, to 1st Nov., 1763, interns received into the house, 329; externs relieved, about 10,000;" whereas the Meath Hospital, which had just then been removed from Meath-street to South Earl-street, received but 130 interns, and 8,004 externs. We presume that this large amount of extern patients arose from the circumstance of the registry having been made from the daily attendance, and not the actual number of individuals who received advice during the year.

The neighbourhood of Francis-street being at that time the most populous and commercial, and to a certain extent the most riotous portion of the city, accidents were of very frequent occurrence there; and to the vast opportunities for studying disease afforded by this Hospital is mainly due the celebrity which Dublin attained as a School of Practical Surgery towards the end of the last century. It was there that the distinguished William Dease made those observations on diseases and injuries which enabled him to produce works which were not only, in point of time, the first surgical writings that emanated from Dublin, but which wrought most useful reforms in the healing art, and are still considered standard in their line. His book of Observations on Wounds of the Head, *published in 1776, was dedicated to "the Governors of the United Hospital of St Nicholas and St Catharine," to which he was then one of the surgeons.*

At the commencement of the present century, the Meath Hospital, which had been constituted by Act of Parliament, in the year 1774, the County of Dublin Infirmary, and which then stood in the Coombe, appears to have been sufficient for the wants of the neighbourhood; and the funds of the Hospital of St Nicholas and St Catharine, derived from voluntary contributions, fell off so much that it was deemed advisable by the Governors to change it to another locality. What became of the early records of the institution is not known, but there still exists "The Governors' Book of the United Hospital of St Mark and St Anne, commencing upon the 2nd of April,

1808," the first entry in which records a meeting of the Medical Governors of the United Hospital of St Nicholas and St Catharine, held in the house in Francis-street upon the above date. The members present were–Messrs Rivers, Doyle, and Hamilton, surgeons; and Drs Burke and Adrien, physicians. This book, in which the transactions of the Hospital Committee were recorded, from the date above specified to the 4th of February, 1832, when the last entry was made, appears to have been entirely the property and solely made use of by the Medical Governors of the institution. Upon the 20th May, in the same year, at a meeting of the Medical Governors, at which, in addition to those already named, Dr Teeling and Mr Fitzsimon were present, it was resolved to move the Hospital to St Mark's Parish, it being no longer necessary where it then stood; to take a lease of a house in Mark-street, for an Hospital, at a rent of £20 a year; and to draw from the funded property of the charity a sum not exceeding £200, to be expended on the new establishment. Upon the 16th September, a meeting was held by the Medical Governors, at the New Infirmary in Mark-street, which was styled "The United Hospital of St Mark and St Anne." The institution was re-opened at No. 15, on the 3rd October. Upon the 5th December a Prospectus was issued, in order to raise subscriptions for the support of the institution. In this it was stated that– "On the expiration of the lease of the house in Francis-street, in the year 1804, the Medical Governors, considering that the West End of the City was amply supplied with similar institutions, richly endowed and well supported, turned their thoughts to this Parish, the only part of the Metropolis that stood in need of such an establishment. Induced by these motives, and strongly encouraged by the inhabitants of that quarter, the Governors opened the Hospital in Mark-street in October last, in a neat and suitable house taken by them, and fitted up with twelve beds, well appointed, for the reception of Medical and Surgical Patients. One Physician, four Surgeons, and an Apothecary, attend each day, from 9 until 11 o'clock, who give advice and medicine to the poor of every description... The Medical Governors, influenced by no principle save that of charity, offer all this to the public, and the use of a fund of ten debentures, with their professional services, without fee or emolument."

Mr Sweetman, of Francis-street, was the Treasurer, and had charge of the fund. During the next six years the Hospital appears to have been in a very languishing condition. Subscriptions were not forthcoming, and the chief entries in the Minute Book during that period concern the election and resignation of several Medical Officers. Some difficulty appearing to exist with respect to the funded money of the charity, it was resolved, on the 23d June, 1815, "to elect Trustees to transfer the property of the institution from the present Treasurer, and to place it in the Bank of Ireland." The five Trustees, who were elected by ballot from among the Medical Governors, were Messrs Callanan, Burke, Adrien, Hamilton, and Fitzsimon. But the fund was not resigned by Mr Sweetman until the year 1822, when he consented to do so, upon the written opinion of Sergeant Lefroy. A copy of this opinion is to be found in the Minute Book already referred to. The Trustees converted the Nine Navigation Debentures, of £100 each, into Four per Cent Government Stock. The Road Debenture not being admissible into the Bank, remained in the hands of Dr Callanan, the Sub-Treasurer.

On the 19th October, 1824, Thomas Rumley, Esq., was elected a Surgeon and Medical Governor of the institution. Subsequently Messrs Brown, Hart, Harrison, Armstrong, Corbet, Brady, Tuomy, and Wall, were elected officers of the institution. With the exception of Mr Rumley, all these officers of the institution forfeited their position, either by death, resignation, or non-attendance. The difficulties of the Hospital having increased, and the entire available fund from interest money and subscriptions not amounting to £50 per annum, a public meeting was held in June, 1829, when it was agreed to remove the institution to the small building formerly a public soup-shop adjoining the Widows' Alms-house, in Mark-street, which was taken from the Churchwardens for that purpose. In the following year, the Hospital was in danger of being closed, from the difficulty of procuring the interest money from the Treasurer and last remaining Trustee. The Medical Governors therefore sought the interference of the Commissioners of Charitable Bequests, who consented to take charge of the fund, and compelled the Treasurer to resign it into their hands. The debts of the Hospital were then cleared off, and the funded money converted into Three-and-a-Half per Cent Stock. The Minute Book of the institution (that alluded to in the foregoing Report) was obtained from Dr Callanan, in February, 1832, by Mr Mathews, the Secretary to the Charitable Bequests' Board, in the keeping of which body it still remains, and after that there is no record of the meetings or proceedings of the institution for several years. For a considerable period subsequent to this, the *institution ceased to exist, the Hospital was closed, and the interest of the funded property in the hands of the Commissioners of Charitable Bequests was employed to liquidate several heavy debts which had accumulated upon it, partly owing to mismanagement, and partly from a defalcation on the part of the Treasurer.*

In July, 1842, Mr Rumley, in connexion with Mr Hamilton, took the house lately occupied as an Hospital in Mark-street from the rector of the parish, re-opened the institution, and supported it for some time from their own private resources. In January, 1843, these gentlemen memorialed the Board of Charitable donations and Bequests, "to direct the interest of the St Mark's Hospital Fund now in their hands to be expended for the benefit of the Hospital, through any channel the commissioners may consider eligible," and at the same time stated that they had expended "£80 in altering and repairing the house, in the purchase of bedding &c., for six intern patients, and in arrangements for the Dispensary," &c. Accordingly, in the February following, the Commissioners made the following order–"That the future dividends be paid to the Incumbent of St Mark's Parish, to be by him paid over to the Medical Attendants of the institution for the time being." Since then, the half-yearly dividend upon £845 17s. 3d., now placed in the Three-and-a-Quarter per Cent Government Stock, and also the interest of the Kinnegad Road Debenture of £50, together amounting to £29 19s. 6d., has been paid over regularly to the Medical Officers of the institution, through the hands of the Incumbent of the Parish, the Rev. George M'Neill.

Although most of the large Hospitals in this City, and the several Infirmaries, Poor-houses, and other institutions in Ireland which afford indoor medical relief, admitted patients labouring under affections of the organs of sight and hearing, there did not, until the commencement of the year 1844, exist in this country any special or distinct hospital for treating such diseases. The want of such an establishment, upon a scale so extensive as to afford any amount of general relief, was long felt by the poor, and generally acknowledged by the upper classes of society. The advantages afforded by such an institution can only be measured by the blessings arising from the perfection of sight and hearing. In the autumn of 1841 Mr Wilde established a Dispensary for Diseases of the Eye and Ear in South Frederick-lane, and supported it for upwards of a twelvemonth, at the end of which time, finding the number of applicants and the consequent expenditure far greater than was originally contemplated, or what could be supported by individual exertion, he determined to try the experiment of making it contribute in part to its own support, by means of a small monthly subscription from those patients whose means enabled them to do so. Paupers have, however, at all times, received advice and medicine gratuitously. The sum paid by each patient is but Sixpence per Month, and this system of partial payments has been found to work exceedingly well. It has produced care, regularity, and attention, and induced a spirit of independence among the lower orders of society worthy of countenance and support; while the annual average sum of £50, received in this way, is in itself a sufficient guarantee to the public and the supporters of the institution, that its benefits are appreciated by the poor, numbers of whom seek its advantages from distant parts of the country. It is true that this partial system of self-support is liable to objections from persons occasionally taking advantage of it for themselves and their children, who are able to pay both for medicine and medical advice; but, on the other hand, the extreme poor reap the advantage of it, and the prescriber and vendor of medicine are alone the losers. Subsequent to this, subscriptions were solicited, and many benevolent individuals came forward to assist the institution. The medical attendance is given gratuitously.

A large majority of patients affected with diseases of the eye, and nearly all those labouring under affections of the ear, only require out-door relief; yet, as several of the most inveterate forms of blindness can be remedied by operation only, and as many of the patients affected with such diseases, or suffering from injuries or violent inflammations, have either come from the country, or live in some of the most wretched and neglected parts of the city, where, from their poverty or the unhealthy condition of their dwellings, they could not possibly obtain those comforts which an hospital affords, it was proposed to establish a special hospital for their reception. In February, 1844, Mr Wilde, having repaid Messrs Hamilton and Brady (the latter being then the representative of Mr Rumley) the sum they expended on the repairs of St Mark's Hospital, was by them given possession of the institution, and appointed its sole Medical Attendant. A Committee of some of the most respectable citizens of Dublin, together with a Secretary and Treasurer, was then formed, in whose hands was placed the fiscal management of the institution, and a presentment was forthwith obtained from the City Grand Jury for a sum equal in amount to that subscribed for the previous half-

year. Since then, the amount of subscriptions have been annually presented for, and the fund belonging to the Hospital has been regularly paid over by the Incumbent of the Parish to the Treasurer, Mr Longfield.

In 1824 several eminent Physicians and Surgeons in Dublin erected the School of Medicine in Park-street–an establishment which soon gained an European and American celebrity, and was for many years one of the chief educational attractions of the city. In 1849 the Proprietors closed the School; and in February, 1850, they disposed of their interest in the premises to Mr Wilde, and the Anatomical and Pathological Collection to the Government for the use of the Queen's Colleges of Cork and Belfast. No building could be better circumstanced for the purposes of an Hospital than this. It has a courtyard in front; is isolated from all surrounding houses, and stands in an enclosed plot of ground, having 61 feet frontage and measuring 95 feet in depth. As stated in the foregoing Report, it has been completely remodelled and fitted up throughout for the purposes of an Ophthalmic Hospital, thereby affording patients advantages which General Hospitals do not admit of. There is a yard to the rere, in which patients can occasionally take exercise; and being in the immediate vicinity of the College Park the institution is remarkably healthy, while the class of affections treated in it secures the inhabitants of the adjoining streets and squares of this most central and respectable part of the Metropolis from any annoyance arising from the introduction of epidemic or infectious diseases. The New Hospital contains 20 beds, and also some accommodation in private wards for the reception of a few pay patients. The money derived from these latter goes to the benefit of the institution. The subsequent history of the institution is contained in the foregoing and previous Annual Reports; and the institution being now upon a more permanent footing than it has ever stood before, it is earnestly to be hoped that the public will appreciate its usefulness, by continuing to afford it sufficient means of support.

APPENDIX B

This memorial was drawn up by the Board of Governors of St Mark's and published in the hospital's fifteenth report, dated 1861-62. It was addressed to the Trustees of a fund established in 1847 by the Society of Friends for famine relief, and sought assistance from the residue of that fund.

"To aid in this good work, the Governors earnestly entreat the assistance of the benevolent of all classes and persuasions." In furtherance of that intention, and knowing that there was a sum of money remaining in the hands of the Society of Friends since the famine period of 1847, the following memorial was addressed to the trustees of that fund by the Board of Governors:–

"GENTLEMEN,–Understanding that a sum of money, subscribed by the people of America for the relief of the suffering poor in Ireland during the famine period of 1846 and 1847, still remains in your hands, and having heard that a portion of it has been already allocated to the relief of the pauper blind, we most earnestly entreat your attention to the circumstances of the Institution of which we are the Governors.

"Ireland has been noted for the number and frequency of the diseases of the eye to which its inhabitants have been liable. This national tendency to blindness was noticed so long ago as the twelfth century.

"Ophthalmia was a prominent item in that lamentable epidemic constitution which formed a portion of the great pathological sequence to the failure of the potato crop, to relieve which the money now in your hands was so generously subscribed by the people of America. In proof of this statement we may mention that 118,835 cases of ophthalmia occurred, in the union workhouses alone, during the four years from 1849 to 1852; and that, when the census was taken in 1851, there was found to be a greater number of blind in Ireland, compared with its population, than in any other country in Europe except Norway, the proportion being 1 totally blind person in every 864 inhabitants.

"In order to meet the exigencies of this state of things there is but one special Ophthalmic Hospital (established in 1844, chiefly by

individual exertion), and which has for the most part been supported by voluntary contributions. Since 1857 it has received annually £100 from Parliament, and the Corporation of the city of Dublin grant it a like sum. The voluntary contributions amount to an average of £114 annually, the Trustees of Bishop Stearne's Charities make it a small grant from year to year, it receives £25 a-year from the Commissioners of Charitable Bequests, and it is partially self-supporting. The total average annual income for the last five years has been £435.

"The number of out-door patients has been, on an average, 2,000 persons for many years past. There are three wards, containing twenty beds, and in these have been treated, during the past five years, on an average 185 persons annually, the great majority of whom were not inhabitants of Dublin or its vicinity, but presented the following provincial proportions:—from Ulster 57; from Munster 152; from Leinster 364; from Connaught 160; besides those from England and Wales.

"The strictest economy has been observed in all the branches of the Institution. Except the Resident Surgeon, none of the medical attendants receive pecuniary remuneration. The result of this on the one hand, and in consequence of the limited accommodation in the Institution on the other, during the last six years the sum of £300 has been capitalized as a reserve fund for the purpose of increasing the hospital accommodation.

"As the wards are generally overcrowded, and as it is considered advisable to have small separate apartments for cases requiring delicate operations on the eye, it is now proposed to increase the hospital accommodation by four new wards, provided a sufficient fund can be raised for building and furnishing such, when it is hoped the public will increase its liberality and provide the means of supporting an additional number of patients.

"Having thus explained the circumstances of the Institution we trust that they will be considered of sufficient importance to induce you to grant a portion of the money at your disposal for this benevolent and national purpose."

That memorial was favourably received by Mr Jonathan Pim and Mr Thomas Bewley, and sanguine expectations were entertained that a sum of money would be granted out of the American fund to enable the Governors to carry out the contemplated improvements. At the public meeting of the Society of Friends, held in Dublin last May, the prayer of the memorial was not granted by the members of that body. Under these disheartening circumstances the Governors determined to effect so much of the proposed improvements as the reserve fund at their disposal should enable them to do, and at the same time to make an appeal to the benevolent to assist them in completing the proposed addition and improvements....

APPENDIX C

The following is taken from the thirteenth report of St Mark's Hospital (1859). Though unsigned, it is written in the first person and is unquestionably the work of Wilde.

The following is a copy of the Memorial presented in September, 1858, to his Excellency the Earl of Eglinton, then Lord Lieutenant, through Lord Naas, Secretary for Ireland, on the subject of making a separate State provision for the Blind:–

"MAY IT PLEASE YOUR EXCELLENCY,

"*As shown by the statistical investigation which I had the honour to submit to your predecessor the Earl of St Germans, contained in one of the Census volumes (on the Status of Disease) recently presented to Parliament, there existed in Ireland, in the year 1851, a greater amount of blind, compared with its population, than any other country in Europe, except Norway, the proportion being one blind person in every 864 inhabitants. The absolute number of persons totally deprived of sight in Ireland, at the time of taking the last Census, was 7,587; and I have reason to believe that the number has increased since then. Of these persons, as many as 995 were in the workhouses at the time specified; but like the other distressed and disabled classes, it is probable that many of them have since come out and mixed with the general population.*

"*Among the most ostensible causes of this calamity may be specified the extreme moisture and variability of our climate at one period of the year, and the harshness and duration of east winds at another; the extreme poverty and inattention to cleanliness of certain classes of the population, the prevalence of rheumatic affections, but above all, the existence of epidemic ophthalmia in the workhouses of Ireland, as a part of the great pestilential constitution which followed in the track of the famine consequent upon the destruction of the potato, during the calamitous period from 1846 to 1852. In proof of this latter assertion, I beg to state to your Excellency, that as shown by the report of the Poor Law Commissioners, 118,835 cases of ophthalmia occurred in the union workhouses alone during the four years from 1849 to 1852. I may also mention, that notwithstanding the greater prevalence of opthalmic diseases in Ireland than other countries, the curriculum of medical education does not require the study of such affections, neither do the Poor Law Commissioners demand any special certificate thereof from the Medical Attendants of workhouses, although the East India and other Boards exact such from their candidates for medical examination. Another cause of the great amount of blind persons in Ireland arises from the number of discharged soldiers, natives of, or resident in the country, who have lost their sight in the public service. By a return received from the military secretary in Ireland, we learn that 106 men were discharged the service in Dublin in one year on account of diseases of the eye.*

"In addition to these existing causes, I may remark that from the earliest period to which our authentic records and annals refer, down to the present time, Ireland has been noted for the number of its blind, as well as for the frequency of outbreaks of epidemic ophthalmia, which have occurred. Upon the circumstances attending these I reported to Parliament in the year 1854. The crowd of persons labouring under diseases of the organs of sight, who flock week by week to St Mark's Ophthalmic Hospital, from all parts of the country, shows that one of the chief endemic diseases of Ireland has not abated either in virulence or distribution.

"To provide suitable treatment for this class of disease, one special hospital exists, where upwards of 2,000 persons are relieved annually as out-door patients, and on an average 150 are treated in the wards of the institution; neither the accommodation of which, nor the funds at the disposal of the Governors, admitting of a greater amount of intern relief.

"To provide for the necessities of the blind in Ireland, who may in round numbers be now taken at 8,000, there are only seven small private asylums, supported solely by the bequests of benevolent individuals, or the voluntary contributions of the charitable, but none of them receive any assistance from the State, or from public taxation. Of these institutions, there are three in Dublin, and one in each of the towns of Belfast, Armagh, Cork, and Limerick; but none of these can with propriety be called a public asylum, even for the limited number it is capable of accommodating. The number of inmates in all these, taken together, averages 150. Some of these asylums receive only those of a certain age, others those of one sex, some those of a particular religion, and others but for a limited

period, and only persons capable of learning certain trades, according to the special objects and intentions of the founders and supporters of each institution. They are each intended for a limited number of a certain class of blind, but neither in their construction, management, nor means of support, are they applicable to the great mass of the pauper blind in this country.

"While the lunatic, the idiotic, the temporary sick, and the criminal have been all amply provided for, partly by the benevolence, and partly owing to the self-interest of mankind, no general public asylums for the pauper blind as yet exist in this country, where irrespective of age, sex, or religion, those of our fellow-creatures, deprived of one of God's greatest blessings, may find shelter, sustenance, clothing, and amusement; and be afforded the means of contributing to their own support, so as eventually to relieve the country of taxation which, whether voluntary or compulsory, is at present supplied for their maintenance.

"Your Excellency is, doubtless, aware, that in almost every country on the Continent a state provision has been made for the blind, and institutions provided where the inmates minister in a great degree to their own happiness, and largely to their support. In England there are several public asylums for the blind, to some of which parochial aid is supplied by the districts from whence the inmates have been received.

"According to the Irish Poor Law Act, 6 & 7 Vict. cap. 92, s. 14, it is enacted, 'That the Guardians of any union may send any destitute person, deaf and dumb, or blind child under the age of eighteen, to any institution for the maintenance of the deaf and dumb, or blind, which may be approved of by the Commissioners, with the consent of the parents or guardians of such child, and may pay the expense of its maintenance there, out of the rates raised under the authority of the said first recited Act.' But as we do not possess any public institution for the blind, irrespective of age, sex, religion, condition of life, capabilities, or limit of period, and as by the Act referred to none of the blind persons over eighteen years of age now in the workhouses could be sent to such institutions even if they did exist, the want of a public asylum adequate to the necessities of the country in this respect must be manifest to your Excellency, and to those who will give the matter serious and charitable consideration.

"Some years ago I brought this matter before the Chief Poor Law Commissioner, but he was then of opinion that the blind would be

better cared and rendered more happy and comfortable by mixing with the seeing population, permanent or floating in the various workhouses. Such, however, I do not believe to be the fact, and it is scarcely just to the blind to have them scattered throughout the workhouses, when by collecting them together, under properly instructed officers, they could be taught industrial arts sufficient to contribute, in part at least, to their own support, and likewise be instructed both in literature and music to an extent that could not be effected in the workhouses.

"In the present improved condition of this country, there is scarcely one other class of the community unprovided for. And I respectfully submit, that tested by the present state of civilization in Europe, the Irish workhouse is not the proper asylum for the pauper blind. Moreover, there are hundreds of blind not in the workhouses, nor admissible to them, who would gladly avail themselves of the benefits of a well-regulated institution.

"I submit to your Excellency's consideration that a soldier, who has spent five or six years in the army, and loses his sight, or has it seriously impaired, either accidentally, or during the discharge of his duty, and who is dismissed with a pension of sixpence a day for nine months, is not a suitable inmate for a workhouse; yet such cases to my own knowledge frequently occur. While I write this I am in communication with Sir Duncan M'Gregor, upon the subject of a well-conducted sub-constable, who after ten years' service in the constabulary force has been dismissed for loss of vision, not consequent on any fault of his own, and with only £22 for his support during the remainder of his life. As soon as that money is spent, this policeman must spend the rest of his life in the workhouse, all his friends having emigrated to America.

"Splendid edifices have been built for the idiotic and insane; and for the education in art, and the benefit of the seeing portion of the population, a national gallery has received a grant from the state. Surely the blind have an equal claim with the former, and a prior one to the latter, upon the resources of the country.

"I respectfully entreat your Excellency to take this national want into your serious consideration, and to recommend such measures to be taken by Her Majesty's Ministers in the ensuing Parliament as shall enable the Poor Law Commissioners, or any other public body, to erect an institution for the maintenance and education of the blind; the cost of the building, and foundation to be levied off the

country at large, and the subsequent support to be contributed by each Poor Law Union, in proportion to the number of inmates from that locality. This will not, I apprehend, in any way interfere with the flow of private benevolence and voluntary contributions towards the existing institutions, nearly all of which have special objects, and some vested funds.

"I can assure your Excellency that such an Institution would be hailed as a great boon by all classes of the community in Ireland, and would largely contribute to that popularity which your Excellency, from your strict sense of justice, as well as your active benevolence, has already acquired.

"The magnitude of the undertaking, and the number of persons to be provided for, prevents any attempt at calling such an institution into existence by means of voluntary contributions. In the event of your Excellency's entertaining this project, I shall be happy to afford those to whom you may intrust the details any information which my observation and experience of the working of such institutions has enabled me to obtain."

APPENDIX D

Staff Listings

NATIONAL EYE AND EAR INFIRMARY

Surgeons

Isaac Ryall	1814-1827	D D Redmond	1879-1891
Richard Morrison	1828-1858	H L Ferguson	1880-1882
J G Hildege	1858-1870	P W Maxwell	1883-1897
H R Swanzy	1871-1897	Louis J Werner	1886-1897
C E Fitzgerald	1871-1897	R K Johnston	1888-1894

Consulting Surgeon

William Colles	1865-1891

Physicians

B Grattan Guinness	1865-1868	John T Banks	1880-1897
J R Kirkpatrick	1869-1880		

Physician for Diseases of the Throat

Richard A Hayes	1881-1897

Consulting Physician

William M Burke	1865-1878

Secretaries

B Grattan Guinness	1865-1868	J G Hildege	1870
J R Kirkpatrick	1869-1870	H R Swanzy	1871-1897

ST MARK'S HOSPITAL

Surgeons

William R Wilde	1844-1876	Arthur H Benson	1879-1897
Henry Wilson	1864-1877	Ferdinand Odevaine	1884-1897
Richard Rainsford	1872-1880	Robert J Montgomery	1894-1897
John B Storey	1877-1897		

Consulting Surgeons

Sir Philip Crampton	1844-1858	John Hamilton	1874-1875
James W Cusack	1858-1860	G H Porter	1875-1894
Robert Adams	1860-1874	E H Bennett	1877-1897

Consulting Physicians

Robert J Graves	1844-1852	Alfred Hudson	1877-1880
William Stokes	1852-1877	James Little	1877-1897

ROYAL VICTORIA EYE AND EAR HOSPITAL

Eye Department
Surgeons

Henry R Swanzy	1897-1913	L B Somerville-Large	1934-1966
C E Fitzgerald	1897-1897	W B Mc Crea	1937-1951
John B Storey	1897-1922	R L Mc Kernan	1943-1965
Arthur H Benson	1897-1912	D H Douglas	1947-1979
P W Maxwell	1897-1917	T J Macdougald	1947-1981
Ferdinand Odevaine	1897-1908	P M Guinan	1947-1981
Louis J Werner	1897-1936	G P Crookes	1951-1981
Robert J Montgomery	1897-1912	T F Roche	1952-1969
Herbert C Mooney	1897-1942	F D McAuley	1962-1984
Frank C Crawley	1900-1935		
Joseph D Cummins	1912-1926	John Blake	1965-
Richard H Matthews	1913-1924	Maurice Fenton	1967-
Euphan M Maxwell	1913-1955	Joseph Walsh	1967-
W C MacFetridge	1919-1934	Alex Tomkin	1969-1984
H B Goulding	1922-1947	L M T Collum	1972-
J B Mc Arevey	1922-1950	David Mooney	1972-
Mary F Connolly	1926-1936	Geraldine Kelly	1978-
Louis E Werner	1925-1965	Hugh Cassidy	1981-
Alan J Mooney	1926-1972	Paul Moriarty	1983-
Harris Tomkin	1928-1980	Peter Barry	1984-
F S Lavery	1928-1965	D McAuliffe Curtin	1984-
		Martin O' Connor	1986-

ENT Department
Physician

Richard Hayes (St Marks from 1879)   1897-1931

Surgeons

T O Graham	1912-1962	Oliver Mc Cullen	1958-1988
L J Curtin	1918-1954	Eric Fenelon	1958-1987
P J Roddy	1925-1966	George Fennell	1967-1989
P D Piel	1926-1958	William Grant	1967-
Margaret Pedlow	1929-1973	Andrew Maguire	1973-
James Hanlon	1935-1951	Michael Walsh	1984-1991
J McAuliffe Curtin	1946-1983	Hugh Burns	1984-
C D O'Connell	1951-1968		

Department of Anaesthetics
Staff Anaesthetists

James Beckett	1914	John Cussen	1953-1957
P A Watson	1914	Sheila Kenny	1950-1973
Silva Deane Oliver	1930-1949	David Hogan	1959-1981
Ruth Campbell	1943-1944	Bee Brennan	1973-1988
Kathleen Bayne	1945-1979	Colette Pegum	1981-
Joseph Woodcock	1946-1951	D D Molyneux	1982-
John Lynham	1949-1980	Anthony P Healy	1982-

Visiting Anaesthetists

Helen Watson	Gerda Johnston
Maeve Curtin	Rohyah Salleh-Dunne

National Ophthalmic Pathology Laboratory of Ireland
Directors

Joan Mullaney	1961-1987	Susan Kennedy	1992-
Michael Farrell	1989-1992		

Department of Radiology
Radiologist

James Griffin   1984-

Hon. Visiting Consultants

Physicians

Sir John Banks	1897-1907	R H Micks	1932-1968
James Little	1897-1911	J G Kirker	1970-
Richard Hayes	1911-1931	A Heffernan	1980-1987

Paediatricians

R Ellsworth Steen	1944-1955	J P R Rees	1964-1986

Surgeons

Edward H Bennett	1897-1906	F J Henry	1944-1948
L G Gunn	1927-1936	J Seton Pringle	1948-1972
J Seton Pringle	1936-1943	David Lane	1984-

Neurological Surgeons

Adams A MacConnell	1936-1973	Christopher Pidgeon	1987-
John P Lanigan	1973-1987		

Plastic Surgeons

A B Clery	1947-1973	M McHugh	1981-

Consulting Aurists

James Hanlon	1951-1959	T O Graham	1965-1966
L J Curtin	1954-1960		

Consulting Oculists

E M Maxwell	1956-1963	H C Mooney	1943-1946

Psychiatrists

H Jocelyn Eustace	1960-1980	Marcus Webb	1981-

Neuro-Ophthalmologists

Alan J Mooney	1926-1972	Peter Eustace	1974-1980

Virologist

Irene Hillary	1977-

Oncologist

Nuala Corcoran	1984-

Facio-Maxillary Surgeons

Niall J Hogan	1952-1984	Frank Brady	1984-

Dental Surgeons

A W W Baker	1897-1924	J E Hogan	1945-1951
G P Moore	1924-1944	Niall J Hogan	1952-1961
Herbert Wright	1945-1956	Edward D Cotter	1961-

Senior Nursing Staff

Matrons from 1897

Miss Wall	⎫ Joint	1897-1903	Miss E M Allen	1932-1957
Miss Hosford	⎭	1897-1908	Miss M C Prunty	1957-1982
Miss A Reeves		1908-1921	Miss A Fitzsimons	1982-
Miss M Power		1921-1932		

Specialised Auxiliary Staff

Almoners/Medical Social Workers from 1938

Dorothy Connor	1938-1947	Maura Reynolds	1956-1961
Nuala O'Duffy	1948-1949	Hilda O'Connell	1971-
Anne Walsh	1950-1956		

Orthoptists from 1946

Heather Siberry-Harris	A Cummins
Sheila Gorevan	Fiona McKee
Brigid Kelly	Patricia Lavery
Alison Petrie	Marion Barrett
Irene Martin	Jennifer Large
W Bernard	Magda Rubalcava
Judith Clarke	Grace Murray
Mary Lou O'Beirne	Nano McCoy
Azra Khan	Tony McAleer
Joan Norman	

Pharmacists from 1955

Mr P Coffey	Mr Seamus Fox
Miss Nancy Flynn	Mrs Maureen Heffernan

Audiometricians

Mrs M Cantwell	Mrs M Glennane
Mrs J Nugent	

Physiotherapist

Mary O'Beirne

Speech Therapists

Miss B Marsh	Mrs P Gillivan-Murphy
Mrs M Gallagher	Ms M Buckley

Medical Photographer

Stephen Travers

Medical Records Officers

Ms Phyllis Tohill	Ms Mairead Lee
Ms Emer Rodgers	

HOSPITAL PERSONNEL — 1992

(Consultant staff excluded)

Council

President

Hon. Mr Justice Frank Griffin

Hon. Treasurer

Mr H J Byrne

Members

Mr J V Arnold	Mr A Maguire
Prof L Collum	Mrs P Maguire
Mrs M Dickson	Mr J McAuliffe-Curtin
The Rt. Hon. the Lord Mayor	Mr J H O'Neill
Alderman Donnelly	Dr J Ruane
Mr M Fenton	Mr J Sherwin
Miss A Fitzsimons	Dr T K Whitaker

Administration

Secretary/Registrar

Mrs Aida Whyte

Accountant

Mr J McKeown

Administrative/Clerical Officers

Mary Ashworth	Sandra King
Margaret Beattie	Ann Maxwell
Devina Brady	Mary Moss
Majella Byrne	Mary Mulligan
Verona Campbell	Noreen McElroy
Dolores Carolan	Colette McCormack
Gwen Cavanagh	Margaret McCormack
Patricia Conn	Terese McCormack
Elva D'arcy	Patricia McSweeney
Edel Doran	Angela O'Brien
Suzanne Gannon	Ann O'Mahony
Fiona Groome	Evelyn Phelan
Susan Holohan	Ann Shiel
Sheena Hoyne	Valerie Teague
Tina Hynes	Amanda Whelan
Adele Jackson	

Telephonists

Marguerette Mitchell	Winston Lindsey

APPENDIX D

Non-Consultant Medical Staff

OPHTHALMOLOGY - PROFESSORIAL UNIT (RCSI)

Clinical Lecturer

Maureen Hillery

Clinical Tutor

A Benedict Smith

Lecturer

Susan Fitzsimmons

OPHTHALMOLOGY - HOSPITAL DEPARTMENT

Senior Registrar

Willam Power

Registrars

Lorraine Cassidy   Conal Hurley
Timothy Horgan

Senior House Officers

John Barrett   Fiona Kearns
Amanda Collum   John Mulhern
John Fenton   Darragh O'Doherty
Michelle Fenton

DEPARTMENT OF OTOLARYNGOLOGY

Senior Registrar

Niall Considine

Registrar

El Gasin El Nagar

Senior House Officers

Mohammed Benamer   Mohammad Sharif
Tat Koh   Salah Widda

DEPARTMENT OF ANAESTHESIA

Registrar

Dr Puri

Chaplains

Catholic: Rev. E Fitzgerald, SJ Lutheran: Pastor G Fritz
C of I: Rev. D Pierpoint   Methodist: Rev. B Griffin
Jewish: Rabbi M Friedberg   Presbyterian: Rev. F Sellar

Nursing and Allied Staff

Matron

Augusta Fitzsimons

Assistant Matron

Elizabeth Phelan

Nurse Tutor

Jean Marie Huet

Administrative Sister

Bridget O'Driscoll

Theatre Sisters

Elizabeth Cleary   Ina Furlong
Alice Finn

Nursing Sisters

Helen Darby   Cora O'Carroll
Noreen Dixon   Annie O'Keeffe
Nora Drumgoole   Noreen Oliver
Veronica Gavin-O'Grady   Maura Reilly
Ann C Murphy   Elizabeth Rigney
Breege Murphy

Staff Nurses

Hazel Argue   Denise Kerley
Maura Bagnall   Ann Leppard
Aileen Bent   Cora Loftus-Flynn
Brigid Bergin   Mary Lynam
Bridget Brady   Daire Mangan
Ann Brophy   Catherine Molloy
Helen Burke   Pauline Moran
Marie Burke   Annette Morgan
Philomena Burke   Maria Morris
Dympna Campbell   Catherine Murphy
Barbara Carolan   Caroline Murphy
Marie Casey   J Murray-Fogarty
Ann Caslin   Catherine McCarthy
Ellen Castles   Mai McCormack
Ann Marie Cochrane   Margaret McDonald
Mary Collopy   Miriam McGrath
Jean Connolly   Linda McGreal

Breda Coyne
Katherina Cribbin
Maureen Cross
Eleanor Crowley
Deirdre Dowling
Bernadette Downes
Pauline Eggleston
Margaret Fitzpatrick
Theresa Flaherty
Dervil Flanagan
Ann Marie Flynn
Bernadette Gavaghan
Sarah Gibbons
Eileen Graham
Siobhan Halpin
Ann Hosty
Aideen Kehoe
Elena Kelly
Theresa Kerins

Gabrielle McKenna
Sarah McMahon
Juliette O'Connor
Mary O'Doherty
C O'Donoghue-Leahy
Ann O'Dwyer
Claire O'Leary
Breda O'Neill
Iris O'Neill
Stephanie O'Neill
Marcella Ormonde
Ann O'Sullivan
Gabrielle O'Sullivan
Mary O'Toole
Ann Power
Ann Prunty
Ann Rooney
Marian Stitt
Annette Ward-McLoughlin

State Enrolled Nurses

Clare Pyne

Agnes Smyth

Nursing Aides

Louise Gorby
Mary Maguire

Ruth McAuliffe-Curtin
Philomena McDonagh

Para-Medical Staff

Medical Social Worker

Hilda O'Connell

Senior Audiologists

Judith Nugent

Mary Glennane

Orthoptists

Nano McCoy (Senior)

Tony McAleer

Physiotherapist

Mary O'Beirne

Radiographers

Marie Blake (Senior)
Louise Bluett

Grainne Rigney
Claire O'Brien

Laboratory Technologists/Technicians

Helen Kavanagh
Paula Devine
Lorraine Maxwell

Marie McGarry
Siobhan O'Keeffe
Damien Tiernan

Senior Pharmacist

Maureen Heffernan

Medical Photographer

Stephen Travers

Phlebotomist

Marie Lucey-O'Connor

Household Staff

Catering Officer

Patricia Gill-O'Grady

Catering Staff

Shane McCarthy
Ann O'Brien

Margaret O'Reilly
Margaret Simmons

Domestic Staff

Joan Allen
Mairead Byrne
Louise Carroll
Pauline Connolly
Breda Cooke
Kathleen Cooke
Maureen Dempsey
Ann Doherty

Kathleen Dowd
Valerie Malone
Lena Monaghan
Mary Morgan
Sharon Quinn
Imelda Reid
Mary Robinson

Head Porter

Gerard McDonnell

Portering Staff

Joseph Armstrong
Christopher Balfe
Christopher Bolton
William Coleman
Paul Connolly
Harry Denby
Thomas Hyland

Patrick Kelly
Thomas Moore
Christopher O'Brien
Patrick O'Callaghan
Hugh O'Keeffe
Paul Woods

BIBLIOGRAPHY

Batchelor, Frederick. 'Hospitals and Hospital Construction' in *The Irish Builder,* Vol 39, p45. Dublin, 1 March 1897.

Cameron, Charles A. *History of the Royal College of Surgeons in Ireland.* Fannin and Co, Dublin, 1916.

Collins, E Treacher. *History and Traditions of Moorfields Eye Hospital.* H K Lewis & Co, London, 1929.

Crowley, Mary F. *A Century of Service, the Story of the Development of Nursing in Ireland.* Dublin, 1980.

Fitzgerald, C E. 'Obituary of Sir Henry Rosborough Swanzy' in *Dublin Journal of Medical Science,* Vol. CXXXV. Dublin, 1913.

Hicks, Frederick G. 'Obituary of Frederick Batchelor' in *Journal of the Royal Institute of Architects of Ireland.* Dublin, 1932

Lindsay, Deirdre. *Dublin's Oldest Charity.* Dublin Anniversary Press, 1990.

McCready, C T. *Dublin Street Names.* Carraig Books, Blackrock, Dublin, 1975 (reprint of 1892 edition).

McDermott M J, and Brioscu A. *Dublin's Architectural Development,* 1800-1925. Tulcamac, Dublin, 1988.

Mitchell, David. *A 'Peculiar' Place the Adelaide Hospital.* Blackwater Press, Dublin, 1989.

Morton, Leslie T. *A Medical Bibliography.* Gower, London, 1983.

Mullaney, Joan. 'The National Ophthalmic Pathology Laboratory and Registry of Ireland' in *Transactions of the Ophthalmological Societies,* Vol 86. London, 1966.

O'Brien, Eoin. *The Charitable Infirmary Jervis Street 1718-1987.* The Anniversary Press, Dublin, 1987.

Slagter, Carien, and Boltendal, Ido. *Met andere ogen....* Utrecht, 1989.

Smyth, Hazel P, Kathleen Lynn. *Dublin Historical Record.* March 1977.

Somerville-Large, L B. 'Dublin's Eye Hospitals' in *Irish Journal of Medical Science,* Nos 225-226. Dublin 1944.

Montgomery Lecture in *Transactions of the Ophthalmological Societies.* London, 1959.

Ophthalmology in Ireland. Guinness, Dublin, 1964.

Somerville-Large, Peter. *Dublin, the First Thousand Years.* Appletree Press, Belfast, 1988.

Swanzy, H R, and Fitzgerald C E. 'Medical Report of the National Eye and Ear Infirmary, Dublin, for 1875' in *Dublin Journal of Medical Science.* Dublin, 1876.

Swanzy, H R. *Handbook on Diseases of the Eye.* London, 1884.

White, T de Vere, *The Parents of Oscar Wilde.* London, 1967.

Wilde, W R. *Narrative of a Voyage.* Curry, Dublin, 1839.

Wilde, W R. *Practical Observations on Aural Surgery.* J Churchill, London, 1853.

Wilson, Denis. *De Iron Trote, the Cork Eye Ear and Throat Hospital.* Eglantine Publications, Cork, 1990.

Wilson, T G. *Victorian Doctor, the Life of Sir William Wilde.* Methuen, London, 1942.

Souvenir Brochure of RVEEH Research Foundation, 5 March 1981.

Souvenir Brochure of Irish Ophthalmological Society, May 1967.

Annual Reports of the National Eye and Ear Hospital, 1865-70.

Annual Reports of the National Eye and Ear Infirmary, 1871-97

Annual Reports of St Mark's Ophthalmic Hospital, 1845-97

Annual Reports of Royal Victoria Eye and Ear Hospital, 1897-1990

Annual Reports of RCSI Department of Ophthalmology, 1987/88/89

INDEX